RECENT ADVANCES
IN ADHESIONS RESEARCH

RECENT ADVANCES IN ADHESIONS RESEARCH

ABIGAIL MCFARLAND
AND
MATTHEW AKINS
EDITORS

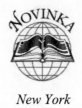

New York

NOTICE TO THE READER

Library of Congress Cataloging-in-Publication Data

Library of Congress Control Number: 2012954192
ISBN: 978-1-62417-447-6

Published by Nova Science Publishers, Inc. †New York

CONTENTS

PREFACE

In this book, the authors present current research in the study of adhesions. Topics discussed in this compilation include surface analysis techniques for root canal filling adhesion studies; polysialylated-neural cell adhesion molecules in the human nervous system at prenatal, postnatal and adult ages; surgical adhesives; interaction of diamond-transition metal substrates and interfacial adhesion enhancement/failure mechanisms; inhibition and impairment of cell adhesions; and effects of anti-cell adhesion molecules to prevent heart transplant rejection.

Chapter 1 – In an effort to solve the problems of clinical failure of endodontic treatments, adhesive materials are used. However, the principles of adhesion in endodontics have several limitations. These limitations are associated with the geometry and the composition/structure of radicular dentin and the various influences of the smear layer produced during chemo-mechanical preparation, irrigants, intra-canal medication, main filling material and endodontic sealers. In endodontics, two interfaces are associated in the adhesion processes, dentin/sealer and sealer/main filling materials. In order to better understand the influence of the irrigant solutions on the dentin and main filling material surfaces, and the effect of these solutions on the adhesion of endodontic sealers to dentin and main filling material, this chapter discusses how surface analysis techniques can be used to evaluate the dentin and main filling material surfaces separately.

Chapter 2 – The polysialylated form of the neural cell adhesion molecule (PSA-NCAM) has received much attention in recent years and it is often used as a marker of neuronal cells undergoing structural and functional changes. The association of NCAM with chains of polysialic acid is finely tuned throughout nervous system development to confer the molecule a role as negative modulator of cell adhesive properties thereby allowing neurons to undergo plastic changes, such as neurite outgrowth and synaptic reorganization, in both embryonic and adult life. In adult mammals, PSA-NCAM expression persists in cerebral regions such as the hippocampus, the olfactory cortex, the medial prefrontal cortex, the amygdala, the hypothalamus, and terminal regions of primary sensory afferents where continuous remodelling has been described. In man, selected populations of central and peripheral neurons have been reported to express PSA-NCAM in normal conditions, supporting the concept of an involvement of this molecule in structural and functional plasticity throughout life. Accordingly, expression of PSA-NCAM is regulated in response to events involving synaptic structural plasticity such as learning, memory consolidation, chronic stress or chronic antidepressant treatment and different types of neuronal lesion models. Interestingly, its localization in subpopulations of primary sensory neurons suggests that PSA-NCAM may also have a part in the processing of somatosensory information. Here, by presenting both original observations from our laboratory and literature data, we review knowledge on the occurrence of the molecule in sensory ganglia, brainstem nuclei and hippocampal formation of the human nervous system at different developmental ages spanning from prenatal and postnatal to adult life. As morphological support of the possible interactions of PSA-NCAM with neurotrophic factors, data on PSA-NCAM codistribution with the neurotrophin BDNF in the brainstem are reviewed and novel findings on PSA-NCAM/BDNF codistribution and colocalization in the hippocampus are presented.

Chapter 3 – A wound may be defined as an injury to any of the body's tissues, especially one caused by physical means and with interruption of continuity. Primary wound healing of a plan-to-plan oriented scar formation is usually accomplished by hand sewing or stapling the corresponding layers of each side of the incision. Both these methods have been associated to wound infection and granule formation due to their degradation in the organism. They also present other disadvantages, such as the need to be removed (in most cases) and the pain associated with their use. As a result of these shortcomings, surgeons have thought of an alternative way: the use of medical tissue adhesives. These adhesives consist on an attractive option to suturing or stapling since they can accomplish other tasks, such as haemostasis and the ability of sealing air leakages and also because they do not represent any risk of needlestick injury to medical staff. Also, the use of an adhesive would reduce the surgeries procedure time since its application presents itself as an easier and faster method to establish tissue adhesion. Despite their advantages, surgical adhesives must obey some clinical requirements. They must hold the two sides of the tissue together until it is no longer necessary, and then they should be degraded to biocompatible products. The most used surgical glues nowadays are the fibrin based adhesives and cyanoacrylates. Fibrin based adhesives present several problems, e.g. immunogenicity and risk of blood transmission diseases such as HIV and BSE. On the other hand, cyanoacrylates have been reported to degrade in aqueous media producing formaldehyde, which causes inflammation and has carcinogenic potential. Other options are now coming into light, and among the synthetic materials, urethane-based adhesives have been considered to be the most promising. These materials may be prepared under the form of pre-polymers (containing free isocyanate groups) and therefore being able to react with amino groups present in the biological molecules establishing adhesion. Another current area of research is the synthesis of UV-curable adhesives. These offer major advantages compared to pre-polymers systems, such as fast-curing rate, control of polymerization heat evolution and are ideal for application to weakened and diseased tissue. Throughout this chapter, examples of currently applied bioadhesives in surgery, as well as their advantages and disadvantages will be described. A special emphasis will be given to the development of polyurethane based adhesives both in the pre-polymer and UV-curable forms.

Chapter 4 – Diamond coating on the conventional transition metal substrates Cr, Fe, Co, Ni, Cu, Ti and their alloys is a promising technology for both structural and functional applications by providing enhanced surface wear/corrosion resistance or thermal conductivity. A major technical barrier so far is that complex interfacial reaction occurs between the gaseous precursors and the substrate components depending on the reactivity, solubility or diffusivity of carbon hydrogen and or oxygen with the metal elements. Especially, the Fe, Co, Ni are strong catalytic elements for preferential formation of non-diamond carbon phases on the substrate surfaces, causing spontaneous spallation of the diamond films once they form. Cu and Ti have no such catalytic effects but mismatch in the thermal expansion coefficient with diamond exists, which also raises severe interfacial adhesion problems. We have performed comprehensive investigations on the diamond deposition on these typical transition metals in terms of nucleation, growth and interfacial bonds, and the adhesion issues are addressed by using high resolution TEM interfacial investigation and synchrotron radiation based analytical technologies. In this chapter, we will introduce our most recent progress in the understanding of diamond-substrate interaction and the mechanism of enhanced interfacial adhesion of diamond coatings on the related substrates.

Chapter 5 – Polysialic acid, an α2,8-sialic acid polymer is specifically bound on the neural cell adhesion molecule (NCAM). PSA binds a significant amount of water molecules and serves as a spacer between cells, inhibiting trans- (NCAM-NCAM) as well as cis-interactions. The PSA expression on neuronal stem cells prevents a premature differentiation of these cells through the inhibition of cell-cell adhesion signaling. Other interactions like integrin-β1 and NCAM on the cell membrane (cis-interaction) are ihnibited through PSA expression. PSA expression on the surface of cells inhibits cell signaling and therefore this sialic acid polymer is responsible for inhibiting premature physiological changes of neuronal stem cells. On the other hand it is also overexpressed on cancer cells, establishing the malignant cell phenotype of these cells. Cancer cell interactions are ihnibited by PSA and therefore these cells do not interact with their environment and keep an „antisocial" state. By PSA overexpression cells do not bind with their environment and can migrate freely through tissues. Stem cell migration is established, as well as migration of cancer cells rendering these cells highly invasive and metastatic.In the present chapter the mecahnism of cell adhesion inhibition through PSA is discussed.

Chapter 6 – Polysialic Acid is a carbohydrate, which binds to the neural cell adhesion molecule NCAM, and contains a high amount of water. It is known that polysialic acid attenuates cell-cell interactions and inhibits differentiation as well as enhances cell migration. Both features are characteristics of highly malignant cancer cells. It has been shown that in a number of highly malignant tumors like glioblastomas, rhabdomyosarcomas, neuroblastomas, and small cell lung cancer, polysialic acid is over-expressed on the surface of these tumor cells. In the present review the possible benefit of polysialic acid overexpression for the tumor cells is discussed, as well as diagnostic and therapeutic strategies towards polysialic acid.

Chapter 7 – Although 100,000 cardiac transplants have been performed, rejection is still a serious problem. Several adhesion molecules play a critical role in the progression of rejection. Recent investigations have proved some promising methodologies targeting cell adhesion molecules for preventing or treating inflammatory diseases.

Although neutralizing antibodies are known to be an effective treatment in cardiovascular diseases, their effect on cardiac transplantation is to be elucidated. In this review article, we described some promising methodologies that use blocking cell adhesion molecules to prevent cardiac rejection.

In: Recent Advances in Adhesions Research   ISBN: 978-1-62417-447-6
Editors: A. McFarland and M. Akins   © 2013 Nova Science Publishers, Inc.

Chapter 1

SURFACE ANALYSIS TECHNIQUES FOR ROOT CANAL FILLING ADHESION STUDIES

Maíra do Prado[1,2] and Renata A. Simão[1]#*

[1]Department of Metallurgic and Materials Engineering, Federa
University of Rio de Janeiro, Rio de Janeiro, RJ, Brazil
[2]Department of Restorative Dentistry - Piracicaba Dental
School - State University of Campinas, Piracicaba, SP, Brazil

ABSTRACT

In an effort to solve the problems of clinical failure of endodontic treatments, adhesive materials are used. However, the principles of adhesion in endodontics have several limitations. These limitations are associated with the geometry and the composition/structure of radicular dentin and the various influences of the smear layer produced during chemo-mechanical preparation, irrigants, intra-canal medication, main filling material and endodontic sealers.

* Maíra do Prado: Department of Metallurgic and Materials Engineering, Federal University of Rio de Janeiro, Av. Athos da Silveira Ramos 149, 21941909, Rio de Janeiro, RJ, Brazil. Department of Restorative Dentistry - Piracicaba Dental School - State University of Campinas, Av. Limeira 901, 13414018, Piracicaba, SP, Brazil.
# Renata A. Simão: Department of Metallurgic and Materials Engineering, Federal University of Rio de Janeiro, Av. Athos da Silveira Ramos 149, 21941909, Rio de Janeiro, RJ, Brazil.

In endodontics, two interfaces are associated in the adhesion processes, dentin/sealer and sealer/main filling materials. In order to better understand the influence of the irrigant solutions on the dentin and main filling material surfaces, and the effect of these solutions on the adhesion of endodontic sealers to dentin and main filling material, this chapter discusses how surface analysis techniques can be used to evaluate the dentin and main filling material surfaces separately.

INTRODUCTION

1. Adhesion in Dentistry

Adhesion can be defined as the ability of dissimilar materials to stick together and not skid or slip under normal conditions of applied loads. Adhesion works both by chemical forces between molecules in close contact as well as mechanical retention. These forces must be sufficient to resist both external loads and internal stresses within deformable bodies.

In dentistry, the theory of bonding was described by Nakabayashi et al. in 1982. The authors described a three-step process that allows hydrophobic restorative materials to adhere to the wet dentin surface. An acid is applied to the dentin surface and rinsed off, for smear layer removal, demineralizing the superficial dentin and exposing the collagen matrix. A resinous material, incorporated in a volatile liquid carrier, such as acetone or alcohol, is then applied to the demineralized dentin. The carrier penetrates the moist dentin surface and carries the resinous material into the collagen matrix and dentinal tubules. The dentin is then air dried to evaporate the carrier, leaving the resinous material behind. The volatile liquid/resinous material is known as the primer. An unfilled or lightly filled resin is then applied to the dentin surface and light cured. This material, known as the adhesive, co-polymerizes with the resin already in the collagen matrix, locking it onto the dentin surface, and providing a hydrophobic surface for co-polymerization with hydrophobic restorative resin materials. The resin infiltrated collagen matrix is known as the hybrid layer (Hansen et al., 1989; Crim, 1990; Erickson, 1992; Van Meerbeek et al., 2003).

Over the years, aiming to simplify the technique, adhesives were developed allowing some steps to be combined. These materials can be classified as two-step etch and rinse or fifth generation; two-step self-etch or sixth generation; and one-step self-etch or seventh generation. These materials all depend on micro-mechanical interlocking from the collagen matrix for retention (Schwartz, 2006).

An important characteristic of dentin bonding is that the dentinal tubules make only a minor contribution to dentin adhesion. Gwinnett (1993) quantified this contribution at 15%. Micromechanical forces from the collagen matrix in the intertubular dentin provide the greater part of the adhesion (Tao and Pashley, 1990; Tagami et al., 1990; Pereira et al., 1999).

2. ADHESION IN ENDODONTICS AND ITS LIMITATIONS

In an effort to solve problems of microbial leakage and clinical failure of endodontic treatments, adhesive materials were introduced in endodontic practice. However, the principles of adhesion in endodontics have several limitations. These limitations are associated with both intrinsic factors, such as the influence of the root canal itself, its geometry and the composition/ structure of radicular dentin, as well as extrinsic factors, such as the influences of the smear layer produced during chemo-mechanical preparation, irrigants, intra-canal medication, the main filling material and endodontic sealers (Schwartz, 2006).

2.1. Influence of the Root Canal

2.1.1. Influence of Root Canal Geometry

The configuration factor or C-Factor, the ratio of bonded to unbonded resin surfaces (Carvalho et al., 1996), is used as a quantitative measurement of the geometry of the cavity preparation for bonding. The greater the percentage of unbonded surfaces, the less stress is placed on the bonded surfaces due to polymerization contraction. Preparations with a favorable geometry have a ratio of approximately 1:1. In the case of root canal system, the ratio might be 100:1 (Carvalho et al., 1996). This occurs because every dentin wall has an opposing wall and there are minimal unbonded surfaces (Schwartz, 2006). According to Yoshikawa et al. (1999), any ratio greater than 3:1 is considered unfavorable for bonding. Because of this unfavorable geometry, it is very hard to achieve a gap-free monoblock in root canal fillings.

Additionally, in the root canal system, due to its shape, the adhesion is different at different depths and the apical third suffers substantial injury. In the apical third, the primer or adhesive application is more difficult, and when the primer is applied, the volatile carrier evaporation is also more difficult due the depth of this area. Paper points are sometimes used for both removal of volatile compounds and primer application.

Nonetheless, acetone or alcohol cannot be effectively removed using paper points, and the primer will not completely spread over all the root surface using this method, adversely affecting the adhesion (Schwartz, 2006). This limitation is clearly observed in the study of Bouillaguet et al. (2003), who reported that lower bond strength values were achieved when bonding in the root canal system than to flat dentin surfaces.

2.1.2. Influence of Dentin Structure

A reduction of dentinal tubules occurs from the cervical to apical thirds in the root canal. The number of dentinal tubules in the apical third is smaller than the number observed in the coronal third (Figure 1).

Consequently, fewer resin tags are formed during the bonding procedures. On the other hand, in this third more intertubular dentin is available for hybridization (Ferrari et al., 2000; Mjor et al., 2001; Mannocci et al., 2004).

The literature indicates that the majority of the retention is provided by micromechanical forces from the collagen matrix in the intertubular dentin (Tao and Pashley, 1990; Tagami et al., 1990; Pereira et al., 1999). If only this aspect were involve in root canal adhesion, the level of adhesion in the apical third might be highest. However, this area is difficult to work with, as already described, and the adhesion problem is much more complicated. Contradictory results are found in the literature: some authors have reported higher bond strengths to dentin in the apical third (Gaston et al., 2001; Mannocci et al., 2004; Muniz et al., 2005), while others have reported lower bond strengths (Yoshiyama et al., 1998; Bouillaguet et al., 2003; Mallmann et al., 2005, Neelakantan et al., 2011), and still others have reported little difference (Burrow et al., 1996; Yoshiyama et al., 1996).

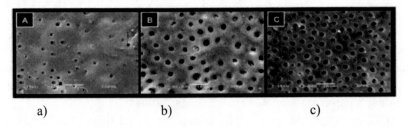

a)   b)   c)

Figure 1. Photomicrographs illustrating the dentinal tubules in the apical (A), middle (B) and cervical (C) thirds.

2.2. Influence of the Smear Layer Produced during Chemo-Mechanical Preparation

During chemo-mechanical preparation, the mechanical action of the instruments produces a layer containing inorganic and organic substances that include fragments of odontoblastic processes, microorganisms and necrotic materials. This layer is called smear layer (Figure 2A).

The smear layer can prevent the penetration of intracanal medications into the dentinal tubules, interfere in the decontamination by irrigant solutions and impede the close contact between root canal filling materials and the root canal walls (Prado et al., 2011). Smear layer removal leads to the opening of the dentin tubules and a cleaner dentin surface (Figure 2B,C), favoring the micromechanical retention in the intertubular dentin and the penetration of sealer in the dentin tubules. Studies show that smear layer removal improves the bonding ability of resin-based sealers and reduces the coronal microleakage (Torabinejad et al., 2002; Neelakantan et al., 2011).

Solutions such as 17% EDTA, 10% citric acid, MTAD or 37% phosphoric acid, applied for different time intervals, are recommended for this purpose. In general, solution application for longer periods allows more efficient smear layer removal and more opened tubules (Prado et al., 2011).

2.3. Influence of Irrigants

The use of different auxiliary chemical substances is essential for successful debridement of root canals during the cleaning and shaping procedures.

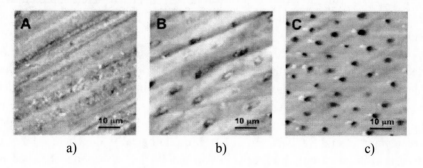

a)   b)   c)

Figure 2. AFM images (50 μm x 50 μm) of smear layer covered dentin surface (A), and after 17% EDTA action for 1 minute (B) and 3 minutes (C).

Sodium hypochlorite has a long history of successful use in endodontics (Vilanova et al., 2012). Three key features make sodium hypochlorite solutions popular among clinicians: the antimicrobial effect and ability to dissolve biofilms (McDonnell and Russell, 1999; Bryce et al., 2009), the capacity to solubilize tissue (Naenni et al., 2004), and the low price and wide availability from many commercial sources (Clarkson and Moule, 1998; Frais et al., 2001). However, this solution is a strong oxidizing agent and leaves behind an oxygen rich layer on the dentin surface that results in increased microleakage (Yiu et al., 2002) and reduced bond strengths (Nikaido et al., 1999; Perdigao et al., 2000; Lai et al., 2001; Morris et al., 2001; Ari et al., 2003; Erdemir et al., 2004; Ozturk et al., 2004). The fact the dentin surface is oxygen rich is probably an important reason for the low bond strengths reported for adhesive resin sealers.

In order to reduce this effect, reducing agents such as ascorbic acid and sodium ascorbate are employed (Moreira et al., 2011; Prasansuttiporn et al., 2011). Other fact to explain the reduced bond strengths is that 5.25% sodium hypochlorite generates collagen degradation and structural disorganization of reminiscent fibrils, which may impede the formation of a consistent hybrid layer (Moreira et al., 2009).

Chlorhexidine has been suggested as an irrigant during root canal therapy based on its antibacterial effects, substantivity and relative absence of cytotoxicity (Jeansonne et al., 1994; Yesilsoy et al., 1995; White et al., 1997). However, this solution is unable to dissolve tissue (Okino et al., 2004). Additionally, chlorhexidine has been suggested as final irrigant (Zehnder, 2006).

In this aspect, Hashem et al. (2009) verified that the bond strength of ActiV GP was improved by using 2% chlorhexidine in the final irrigation after 17% EDTA. Additionally, chlorhexidine is a matrix metalloproteinases (MMP) inhibitor that can arrest degradation of the hybrid layer in vivo (Hebling et al., 2005).

Studies have evaluated the association between NaOCl during chemo-mechanical preparation with 2% chlorhexidine as final irrigant, observing that this association leads to the formation of byproducts, forming what is called the chemical smear layer, which covers the dentin surface and can interfere in the adhesion process (Vivacqua-Gomes et al., 2002; Bui et al., 2008; Krishnamurthy and Sudhakaran, 2010). Morphologically, the chemical smear layer is different from the mechanical smear layer, as can be observed in Figure 3. The mechanical smear layer is flatter and regular while the chemical smear layer has a more irregular surface that looks like a flower or starfish.

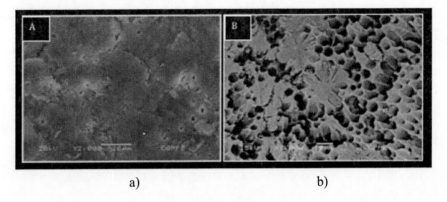

a)   b)

Figure 3. Mechanical (A) and chemical (B) smear layer.

As observed, the different irrigant solutions used in root canal treatment can positively or negatively affect the adhesion of root canal fillings to dentin.

2.4. Influence of Intra-Canal Medication

One of the major factors associated with endodontic failure is the persistence of microbial infection in the root canal system and periradicular area (Nair et al., 1990). Intra-canal medication tends to be effective against microorganisms that have resisted the root canal preparation. Besides this, medicines control persistent exudation and the destructive action of osteoclasts present in external dental resorption (Estrela et al., 1995; Gomes et al., 2006).

Currently, the material with the most scientific and popular support for use as an intra-canal medicament is calcium hydroxide. Calcium hydroxide has been used in dentistry for over 40 years in a variety of applications, such as pulp capping and apexification. When used as an intra-canal medication, calcium hydroxide powder can be mixed with sterile water, saline, anesthetic or chlorhexidine. Also, a commercial preparation of calcium hydroxide can be used (Gomes et al., 2006; Farhad et al., 2012).

Calcium hydroxide is believed to have many of the properties of an ideal root medication. For calcium hydroxide to act effectively as an intracanal medication, it should ideally occupy all the pulp space, thereby diffusing into areas inaccessible to instruments. Its effectiveness is linked to the diffusion of hydroxyl ions through the dentinal tubules and accessory canals into areas where bacteria and their byproducts may be harbored. In addition to acting as a physical barrier, the calcium hydroxide dressing can both prevent root canal re-infection and interrupt the nutrient supply to the remaining bacteria (Gomes et al., 2006).

However, studies show that calcium hydroxide cannot be completely remove from the root canal system before obturation and that the residual calcium hydroxide paste can act as a physical barrier, possibly preventing effective bonding in some areas. Additionally, the high pH can act to neutralize the acid primer in self-etching adhesives (Lambrianidis et al., 1999; Kim et al., 2002; Sevimay et al., 2004; Schwartz, 2006).

2.5. Influence of the Main Filling Material

The obturation step of root canal preparation consists of the use of a main filling material associated with an endodontic sealer. Regarding the main filling material, gutta-percha cones are at present the most commonly used material. They are biocompatible, dimensionally stable, radiopaque and thermoplastic (Gomes et al., 2007). Gutta-percha cones are composed of organic components (gutta-percha polymer and wax/resins) and inorganic ones (zinc oxide and barium sulphate). Small percentages of coloring agents and antioxidants can also be present (Spangberg, 1998; Gurgel-Filho et al., 2003). Although gutta-percha cones are the most commonly used material, they do not have bondability characteristics, i.e., the cones do not adhere to the endodontic sealer.

To increase the adhesion between gutta-percha cones and endodontic sealers, a gutta-percha polybutadiene-diisocyanate-methacylate resin-coating was suggested. However, Tay et al. (2005) reported that gaps and leakage were identified between the gutta-percha resin-coating and the sealer.

Resilon is a synthetic thermoplastic polymer based on polymers of polyester containing bioactive glass and radiopaque fillers. The filler content is approximately 65% by weight. Resilon works like gutta-percha and is available in the same variety of master cones and accessory cones. Also, Resilon pellets are available to use in backfilling with thermoplasticized techniques. Thus, Resilon can be used in the same obturation techniques as gutta-percha. Resilon is associated with the use of Epiphany, Real Seal, Epiphany SE and Real Seal SE sealers (Kim et al., 2010).

The bondability of Resilon with these sealers is attributed to the incorporation of methacrylate-based resin components (Tay et al., 2006). The manufacturer claimed the Resilon system forms a monoblock. However, over the years, studies have shown there is not complete adhesion between the interfaces and the monoblock formation is not complete.

Gutta-percha and Resilon cones are manufactured under aseptic conditions, but they can be contaminated by handling, aerosols and physical sources during the storage process. Because of their thermoplastic characteristics, conventional heating processes cannot be used for sterilization (Gomes et al., 2007). Chemical substances such as sodium hypochlorite and chlorhexidine are therefore used for cone disinfection (Cardoso et al., 1999, Gomes et al., 2005; Royal et al., 2007), but they can alter the surface of these materials (Valois et al., 2005; Isci et al., 2006; Prado et al., 2012).

2.6. Influence of Endodontic Sealers

To provide a fluid-tight seal of the canal space, a sealer is required along with the main filling material. The sealer fills the spaces not occupied by the main filling material, such as irregularities on the dentin surface, grooves and ramifications. For this reason, the sealer has as much or more importance than the main filling material in providing a successful clinical outcome (Gatewood, 2007). The sealers are divided into four major groups: zinc oxide–eugenol–based sealers, calcium hydroxide-based sealers, glass-ionomer sealers and resin-based sealers. This chapter focuses on resin-based endodontic sealers.

The resin-based endodontic sealers are divided into two groups: epoxy resin-based sealers and methacrylate resin-based sealers.

The epoxy resin sealer, named AH Plus, shows good handling characteristics and adhesion to dentin (Limkangwalmongkol et al., 1991), but significant toxicity in the unset state (Spangberg, 1969). However, after 24 hours, the epoxy sealer has one of the lowest toxicities of all endodontic sealers (Wennberg and Ørstavik , 1990). The good adhesion to dentin can be attributed to the fact that AH Plus (Dentsply, Petropolis, RJ, Brazil) is based on the polymerization reaction of epoxy resin–amines and has excellent physical properties and less volumetric polymerization shrinkage (Vilanova et al., 2012).

The methacrylate resin-based sealers are represented by two systems: EndoREZ (Ultradent Products Inc, South Jordan, UT, US) and RealSeal (Sybron Dental Specialties, Orange, CA, US).

EndoREZ is a hydrophilic, two-component (base and catalysts), dual-curing self-priming sealer. This sealer can be used with gutta-percha or with resin-coated gutta-percha cones, the latter with the objective of establishing continuous adhesion (uniblock or monoblock) between all materials. The sealer is supplied in a double barrel auto-mixing and delivery syringe and meets the basic requirements of an endodontic sealer. The manufacturer recommends that after preparation, the root canal walls should remain slightly moist to take maximum advantage of the hydrophilic properties of the sealer, thus allowing for resin tags to penetrate into the dentinal tubules, and the formation of a hybrid layer with the collagen fiber network. However, too much water can cause water permeation during the polymerization process and result in the entrapment of water droplets in the sealer, resulting in bond disruption and an increase in leakage. Also, EndoREZ is associated with gap formation resulting from polymerization shrinkage (Schwartz, 2006).

Real Seal or Epiphany is a dual-cure sealer, composed of urethane dimethacrylate (UDMA), poly dimethacrylate (PEGDMA), ethoxylated bisphenol A dimethacrylate (EBPADMA) and bisphenol A glycidyl methacrylate (BIS-GMA), barium borosilicate, barium sulfate ($BaSO_4$), bismuth oxychloride, calcium hydroxide, photo initiators, and a thinning resin. In addition, the system comes with a self-etching primer. Real Seal SE or Epiphany SE has the same composition, but the primer is introduced in the sealer and is a compound. When this product was developed, monoblock formation was promised, that is, the primer would form a hybrid layer with dentin, bonding to the sealer, and then bonding to the Resilon core. However, this was not borne out in practice.

In fact, several studies have shown that methacrylate resin-based sealers are worse than epoxy resin-based sealers in terms of bond strength. This can be explained because methacrylate resin-based sealers undergo incomplete polymerization inside the root canal and significant volumetric shrinkage during polymerization. Additionally, the high C-factor value of the canal causes accentuated interfacial gap formation (De-Deus et al., 2009; Vilanova et al., 2012).

3. TECHNIQUES COMMONLY USED FOR ADHESION ANALYSIS

Adhesive materials are frequently compared using bond strength and microleakage tests (Hashem et al., 2009; Jacobovitz et al., 2009; Hirai et al., 2010; Shokouhinejad et al., 2010; Neelakantan et al., 2011). Bond strength refers to the force per unit area required to break the bond between the adhesive material and dentin. It is usually described in Mega Pascal units (MPa), that is, Newtons per square millimeter. A good obturation material is one that is effective in preventing microleakage and, in some cases, bond strength may not be the major factor for defining the best system for use in each application. When adhesion studies in endodontics are performed, it is important keep in mind that there are two interfaces that must be investigated: the dentin/sealer and sealer/main filling material interfaces. To better understand the influence of the irrigant solutions on the formation of these two interfaces, surface analysis techniques have been used to evaluate the effect of the solutions on the dentin and main filling material surfaces separately.

4. SURFACE TECHNIQUES USED FOR ADHESION ANALYSIS

Scanning electron microscopy (SEM), contact angle measurement and atomic force microscopy (AFM) have been employed in studies of the influence of different irrigants used during endodontic treatment on the dentin and main filling material surfaces. Both physical and chemical effects are examined, as discussed below.

4.1. Scanning Electron Microscopy

The scanning electron microscope uses a focused beam of high-energy electrons to generate a variety of processes at the surface of specimens. Different signals that derive from electron-sample interactions can be detected and reveal information about the sample, including surface morphology and chemical composition. In most applications, secondary electrons emanating from the sample are collected over a selected area of the surface and a two-dimensional image is generated that displays spatial variations in height within this area.

Areas ranging from approximately centimeters to microns in size can be imaged using conventional SEM techniques (magnification ranging from 20X up to 100,000X). X-rays are also generated by the interaction of the electron beam with the sample, making it possible to perform chemical analysis of selected areas. This approach is especially useful in qualitatively or semi-quantitatively determining and mapping the chemical composition of the sample. This procedure is known as energy dispersive spectroscopy (EDS).

SEM operation consists of an emitting filament located in a vacuum environment. The electrons are guided to the sample by a series of electromagnetic lenses in the electron column. The resolution and depth of field of the image are determined by the beam current and the final spot size, which are adjusted with one or more condenser lenses. The lenses are also used to correct the beam shape in order to minimize the effects of spherical aberration, chromatic aberration, diffraction, and astigmatism. The electrons interact with the sample within a few nanometers to several microns of the surface, depending on beam parameters and sample type. Electrons are emitted from the sample primarily as either backscattered electrons or secondary electrons. Secondary electrons are the most common signal used for investigation of surface morphology. They are produced as a result of interactions between the primary beam electrons and weakly bounded electrons in the conduction band of the sample. Some energy from the beam electrons is transferred to the conduction band electrons in the sample, providing enough energy for them to escape from the sample surface as secondary electrons. Secondary electrons are low-energy electrons (<50eV), so only those formed within the first few nanometers of the sample surface have enough energy to escape and be detected. High-energy beam electrons that are scattered back out of the sample (backscattered electrons) can also form secondary electrons when they leave the surface. Since these electrons travel further into the sample than the secondary electrons, they can emerge from the sample at a much larger distance from the impact of the incident beam, which makes their spatial distribution larger. Once these electrons escape from the sample surface, they are typically detected by an Everhart-Thornley scintillator photomultiplier detector. The SEM image formed is the result of the intensity of the secondary electron emission from the sample at each x,y data point during the scanning of the electron beam across the surface.

Along with the secondary electron emission used to form a morphological image of the surface in SEM, a number of other signals are emitted as a result of the electron beam impinging on the surface. Each of these signals carries information about the sample, providing clues about its composition. Two of the most commonly used signals for investigating composition are x-rays and backscattered electrons. X-ray signals are commonly used to provide elemental analysis by the attachment of an energy-dispersive spectrometer (EDS) or wavelength-dispersive spectrometer (WDS) to the SEM system. X-ray emission results from inelastic scattering between the beam electrons and the electrons of the sample atoms. This interaction results in the ejection of an inner shell electron from the atom, creating a void that is filled by an outer shell electron. This jump from an outer to inner shell results in a change in energy that produces either an X-ray or an Auger electron. The emitted X-ray has energy equal to the difference in energy between the involved levels, carrying information about the chemical nature of the atom from which it was emitted. . The X-rays are then detected by either a lithium-drifted silicon detector for an EDS system, or a gas proportional counter detector for a WDS system. In this way, an X-ray spectrum collected with an EDS system is generated (Davis, 1997; Voutou and Stefanaki, 2008).

4.1.1. The Use of SEM to Evaluate the Dentin Surface

The first study using SEM for this purpose date from 1975, when McComb and Smith for the first time observed the smear layer. After that, Mader et al. (1984) characterized this layer. This layer can be observed in the frontal plane to the dentinal tubule and is thin, irregular, granular, fragile and poorly adhered to the root canal surface layer, being approximately 1 to 5 μm thick. Additionally, when observed in lateral plan, this layer can also be compressed up to 40 μm inside the dentine tubules during preparation. These features are called "smear plug". Studies performed to evaluate the effect of this layer on the adhesion have concluded that this layer can be removed using chelating or acid agents.

EDTA and citric acid are the most employed solutions for root canal smear layer removal, while 37% phosphoric acid is the best solution for coronal smear layer removal. In 2011, Prado et al. proposed the use of 37% phosphoric acid for root canal smear layer removal in gel formulation, used on coronal surface as well as solution formulation. The two formulations were evaluated due to the shape of the root canal and the already discussed difficulties found regarding penetration and removal of the gel inside the root canal. Since EDTA and citric acid are commonly employed for this purpose, the phosphoric acid action was compared with the two last solutions in time periods of 30 seconds, 1 minute and 3 minutes. The study evaluated the degree of smear layer removal and a scoring system (Figure 4) was used: score 1 = no smear layer, with all tubules cleaned and opened; score 2 = few areas covered by smear layer, with most tubules cleaned and opened; score 3 = smear layer covering almost all the surface, with few tubules opened; and score 4 = smear layer covering all the surface.

Prado et al. (2011) showed that none of the substances analyzed was effective for removal of the smear layer after 30 seconds. After 3 minutes, all the substances worked well in the middle and cervical thirds, with phosphoric acid solution exhibiting excellent results even in the apical third.

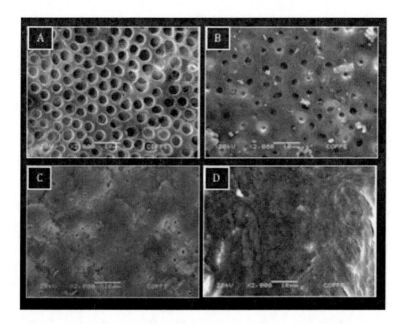

Figure 4. Representative images of scores 1 (A), 2 (B), 3 (C) and 4 (D).

The use of phosphoric acid gel is not indicated because although phosphoric acid gel has shown good results, the persistence of a residual layer of this substance in some samples was observed, mainly in the apical third. A final wash with 5mL of distilled water was not able to remove the gel existing in the apical area. The findings of the study indicate that phosphoric acid solution may be a promising agent for radicular smear layer removal.

4.1.2. The Use of SEM to Evaluate Filling Material Surfaces

The prevention of contamination of the root canal system is an important aspect of endodontic therapy. Gutta-percha and Resilon are used for obturation of the root canal system. Although these materials are manufactured under aseptic conditions, they can be contaminated by handling, aerosols, and physical sources during the storage process. Because of their thermoplastic characteristics, conventional processes using moist or dry heat cannot sterilize them. Therefore, rapid chair-side chemical disinfection is needed. Sodium hypochlorite (NaOCl), chlorhexidine (CHX), and MTAD have been used for this purpose. In 2003, Short et al. used SEM to evaluate the effect of NaOCl on the surface of gutta-percha cones and observed that after disinfection, gutta-percha should be rinsed in alcohol or distilled water to remove the crystallized NaOCl before obturation. In addition, the authors mentioned that that presence of NaOCl crystals on the cone impair the obturation seal.

Gomes et al. (2007), using SEM, evaluated the effect of chlorhexidine and NaOCl on the surface of gutta-percha and Resilon cones after rinsing. They found that these solutions did not cause changes in the surface of these materials. However, there was a lack in the literature regarding two main questions: (1) the effect of MTAD on surfaces and (2) if there is a need to perform a final rinse step after all the solutions. To answer these questions, in 2011 Prado et al. published a paper evaluating the effect of NaOCl, CHX and MTAD on gutta-percha and Resilon surfaces with and without a final rinse using SEM and EDS analysis. The results indicated that with the use of NaOCl without rinse, there was chloride crystal formation in all samples (Figure 5A). When the cones were rinsed, the crystals were removed. When 2% chlorhexidine was used, no change was observed. MTAD without rinse showed the presence of a precipitate in gutta-percha cones (Figure 5B). When the cones were rinsed, this was eliminated.

The authors concluded that the final rinse is essential, especially when NaOCl and MTAD are used in the cone disinfection process (Prado et al., 2011).

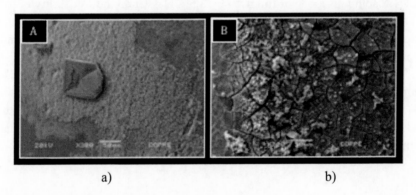

a)   b)

Figure 5. Surface of gutta-percha cones after the use of NaOCl (A) and MTAD (B) without a final rinse.

4.2. Contact Angle Measurement

The contact angle is a measure of the ability of a liquid to spread on a surface. The method consists of measuring the angle (θ) between the outline tangent of a drop deposited on a solid and the surface of this solid (Figure 6).

The contact angles give information on two aspects: the affinity of a liquid to a solid surface (wettability) and the surface free energy of the solid when more than one liquid is used. A drop with a contact angle over 90° indicates poor wetting, poor adhesiveness and low surface free energy. A drop with a small contact angle reflects better wetting, better adhesiveness and higher surface energy (Ramé-Hart Instrument Co.).

This technique has been used in endodontics to evaluate irrigant solutions and medicines in relation to surface free energy of dentin and main filling materials and wettability of sealers on dentin and main filling material surfaces. Nakashima and Terata (2005) proposed the use of 3% EDTA for smear layer removal because according with their study, the contact angle between the endodontic sealer solution (including eugenol, non-eugenol, polycarboxylic acid and resin sealers) and dentin decreased in the 3% EDTA groups but increased when 15% EDTA was used for the same purpose.

Later, Dogan Buzoglu et al. (2007) evaluated the effects of combined and single use of EDTA, RC-Prep and NaOCl on the surface free energy of canal wall dentine and observed that the of chelating agents alone or in combination with NaOCl decreased the wettability of the root canal wall dentine.

However, Yılmaz et al. (2011) evaluated the effect EDTA, EDTA-T and REDTA solutions alone or followed by 2.5% NaOCl on the wettability of root canal dentin and observed that combined and single use of experimental solutions and NaOCl significantly decreased the water contact angle and increased the surface free energy of the root canal dentin.

In 2011, Prado et al. evaluated the surface free energy of the two main filling materials, gutta-percha and Resilon, after disinfection procedures using 2% chlorhexidine and 5.25% NaOCl and the wettability of AH Plus endodontic sealers in contact with gutta-percha and Real Seal SE in contact with Resilon surfaces.

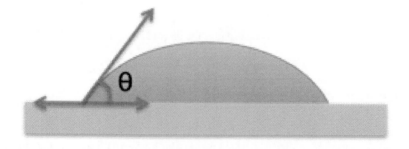

Figure 6. Contact angle measurement (θ).

The authors observed that when disinfectant solutions were used, the surface free energy of main filling materials was higher. Regarding the interaction between materials and sealers, the use of chlorhexidine showed lower values of contact angle, followed by NaOCl.

In the same year, De Assis et al. investigated the wettability of two endodontic sealers, AH Plus and Real Seal SE, in contact with dentine treated with 5.25% sodium hypochlorite and 2% chlorhexidine in the presence or absence of a smear layer. The authors observed that smear layer removal and final flush with chlorhexidine favor the wettability of the AH Plus and Real Seal SE sealers.

4.3. Atomic Force Microscopy

Atomic force microscopy (AFM) consists of scanning a sharp tip on the end of a flexible cantilever across a sample surface while maintaining a small, constant force. The tips typically have an end radius of 2nm to 20nm, depending on type. The scanning motion is conducted by a piezoelectric tube scanner, which scans the tip in a raster pattern with respect to the sample (or scans the sample with respect to the tip). The tip-sample interaction is monitored by reflecting a laser off the back of the cantilever into a split photodiode detector. By detecting the difference in the photodetector output voltages, changes in the cantilever deflection or oscillation amplitude are determined. The two most commonly used modes of operation are contact mode AFM and tapping mode AFM, which are conducted in air or liquid environments (Vilalta-Clemente and Gloystein, 2008).

Contact mode AFM consists of scanning the probe across a sample surface while monitoring the change in cantilever deflection with the split photodiode detector. A feedback loop maintains a constant force, in turn maintaining a constant cantilever deflection by vertically moving the scanner to maintain a constant photodetector difference signal. The distance the scanner moves vertically at each x,y data point is stored by the computer to form the topographic image of the sample surface. Typically, forces range between 0.1 and 100nN (Analytical Instrumentation Facility/Digital Instruments/Veeco Metrology).

AFM generates hree-dimensional images, provides information about surface roughness and can be used to determine chemical and mechanical properties such as adhesion, elasticity, hardness and rupture bond lengths (Cappella and Dietler, 1999).

In endodontics, AFM has been used to evaluate the main filling material and the effect of decontaminant solutions on its surfaces and to evaluate the effect of irrigant solutions in dentin surface, both by topographic images. Additionally, AFM has been used to evaluate the adhesion between dentin surface/sealer and mail filling material/sealer by using force curve analyses.

In 2004, Valois et al. investigated the topography of four commercially available standardized gutta-percha cones with atomic force microscopy. The next year, the same group compared the effects of 2% chlorhexidine and 5.25% sodium hypochlorite on gutta-percha cones by AFM. The authors examined 12 different regions of the cone and the root mean square was measured. They observed there was no deterioration in the topography when chlorhexidine was used. However, the RMS parameter for topography increased after 10 min of 5.25% NaOCl exposure.

Isci et al. (2006) evaluated the effects of 2% chlorhexidine and 5.25% sodium hypochlorite on Resilon cones by AFM. The authors examined seven regions of the cone and root mean square was measured. They concluded that sodium hypochlorite and chlorhexidine solutions significantly decreased the RMS values of Resilon cones with 5-min applications.

In 2012, Prado et al. performed the same analyses to evaluate the effects of 2% chlorhexidine and 5.25% sodium hypochlorite on gutta-percha and Resilon cones by AFM. However, unlike Valois et al. and Isci et al., the same area of the same cone was evaluated in different periods of time. The authors observed that the use of 5.25% NaOCl is associated with local changes in surface roughness of gutta-percha cones. No change was observed when chlorhexidine was used. However, different from Isci et al., the use of all tested solutions did not produce any changes in the Resilon surface.

Also related to the effect of 2% chlorhexidine and 5.25% sodium hypochlorite on gutta-percha and Resilon cones, De Assis et al. investigated the adhesion force (Fad) between root canal sealers and gutta-percha and Resilon cones after the use of chlorhexidine and sodium hypochlorite. For this purpose, AFM tips containing AH Plus sealer were used to obtain force vs. distance curves regarding gutta-percha surfaces and AFM tips containing Real Seal SE sealer were used to obtain force vs. distance curves regarding Resilon surfaces. Fad was calculated from the force curves.

The authors concluded that the decontamination of gutta-percha and Resilon with 2% chlorhexidine resulted in higher Fad values. The use of CHX in the disinfection process of gutta-percha and Resilon cones may be a better option before root canal obturation. Regarding dentin surface, in 2006, De-Deus et al. examined changes of dentine surfaces during demineralization with EDTA, EDTAC and citric acid, using a liquid cell during AFM analyses, in real-time. The authors concluded that the method developed for real-time observation of dentine surfaces is valuable to evaluate demineralization and that the most effective demineralizing substance was citric acid.

In 2012, Prado et al. compared the smear layer removal using scanning electronic microscopy and atomic force microscopy. The authors observed that when AFM images were analyzed, a thicker smear layer and fewer opening tubules were observed compared to the SEM images. They concluded that AFM topographic analysis, as well as phase contrast images, are by far the best methods to detect the presence of smear layer compared to SEM.

CONCLUSION

The use of techniques to analyze the surfaces involved in the adhesion process in endodontics is helpful to elucidate the action of the irrigant solutions commonly used in endodontic practice in its interfaces (dentin/sealer and sealer/main filling material). This information can be useful to improve the bonding strength and reduce coronal microleakage of root canal fillings.

REFERENCES

Ari, H.; Yasar, E.; Belli, S. Effects of NaOCl on bond strengths of resin cements to root canal dentin. *J. Endod.*, 2003, 29, 248 –51.

Bayne, S. C.; Thompson, J. Y.; Swift Jr, E. J.; Stamatiades, P.; Wilkerson, M. A characterization of first-generation flowable composites. *J. Am. Dent. Assoc.*, 1998, 129, 567–77.

Bouillaguet, S.; Troesch, S.; Wataha, J. C.; Krejci, I.; Meyer, J. M.; Pashley, D. H. Microtensile bond strength between adhesive cements and root canal dentin. *Dent. Mater.*, 2003, 19, 199 –205.

Bouillaguet, S.; Troesch, S.; Wataha, J. C.; Krejci, I.; Meyer, J. M.; Pashley, D. H. Microtensile bond strength between adhesive cements and root canal dentin. *Dent. Mater.*, 2003, 19, 199 –205.

Bryce, G.; O'Donnell, D.; Ready, D.; Ng, Y. L.; Pratten, J.; Gulabivala, K. Contemporary root canal irrigants are able to disrupt and eradicate single- and dual-species biofilms. *J. Endod.*, 2009, 35, 1243–8.

Bui, T.; Baumgartner, J.; Mitchell, J. Evaluation of the interaction between sodium hypochlorite and chlorhexidine gluconate and its effect on root dentin. *J. Endod.,* 2008, 34, 181–5.

Burrow, M. F.; Sano, H.; Nakajima, M.; Harada, N.; Tagami, J. Bond strength to crown and root dentin. *Am. J. Dent.,* 1996, 9, 223–9.

Cappella, B.; Dietler, G. Force-distance curves by atomic force microscopy. *Surface Science Reports*, 1999, 34, 1-104

Cardoso, C. L.; Kotaka, C. R.; Redimersky, R.; Guilhermetti, M.; Queiroz, A. F. Rapid decontamination of gutta-percha cones with sodium hypochlorite. *J. Endod.*, 1999, 25, 498–51.

Carvalho, R. M.; Pereira, J. C.; Yoshiyama, M.; Pashley, D. H. A review of polymerization contraction: the influence of stress development versus stress relief. *Oper. Dent.*, 1996, 21, 17–24.

Clarkson, R.; Moule, A. Sodium hypochlorite and its use as an endodontic irrigant. *Aust. Dent. J.,* 1998, 43, 250–6.

Crim, G. A. Prepolymerization of Gluma 4 sealer: effect on bonding. *Am. J. Dent.,* 1990, 3, 25–7.

Davis, U. C. (1997). Introduction to the Scanning Electron Microscope: Theory, Practice, and Procedures. Available from: URL: https://imf. ucmerced.edu/downloads/semmanual.pdf

De Assis, D. F.; do Prado, M.; Simão, R. A. Effect of disinfection solutions on the adhesion force of root canal filling materials. *J. Endod.,* 2012, 38, 853-5.

De Assis, D. F.; do Prado, M.; Simão, R. A. Evaluation of the interaction between endodontic sealers and dentin treated with different irrigant solutions. *J. Endod.,* 2011, 37, 1550-2.

De-Deus, G.; Di Giorgi, K.; Fidel, S.; Fidel, R. A.; Paciornik, S. Push-out bond strength of Resilon/Epiphany and Resilon/Epiphany self-etch to root dentin. *J. Endod.,* 2009, 35, 1048-50.

De-Deus, G.; Paciornik, S.; Pinho Mauricio M. H.; Prioli, R. Real-time atomic force microscopy of root dentine during demineralization when subjected to chelating agents. *Int. Endod. J.,* 2006, 39, 683-92.

Dogan Buzoglu, H.; Calt, S.; Gümüsderelioglu, M. Evaluation of the surface free energy on root canal dentine walls treated with chelating agents and NaOCl. *Int. Endod. J.*, 2007, 40, 18-24.

Erdemir, A.; Ari, H.; Gungunes, H.; Belli, S. Effect of medications for root canal treatment on bonding to root canal dentin. *J. Endod.,* 2004, 30, 113– 6.

Erickson, R. L. Surface interactions of dentin adhesive materials. *Oper. Dent.*, 1992, Suppl. 5, 81–3.

Estrela, C.; Sydney, G. B.; Pesce, H. F.; Felippe Jr, O. Dentinal diffusion of hydroxyl ions of various $Ca(OH)_2$ pastes. *Braz. Dent. J.*, 1995, 6, 5-9.

Farhad, A. R.; Barekatain, B.; Allameh, M.; Narimani, T. Evaluation of the antibacterial effect of calcium hydroxide in combination with three different vehicles: An in vitro study. *Dent. Res. J.* (Isfahan). 2012 Mar.-Apr.; 9(2): 167–172.

Ferrari, M.; Mannocci, F.; Vichi, A.; Cagidiaco, M. C.; Mjor, I. A. Bonding to root canal: structural characteristics of the substrate. *Am. J. Dent.*, 2000, 13, 255– 60.

Frais, S.; Ng, Y.; Gulabivala, K. Some factors affecting the concentration of available chlorine in commercial sources of sodium hypochlorite. *Int. Endod. J.* 2001, 34, 206–15.

Gaston, B. A.; West, L. A.; Liewehr, F. R.; Fernandes, C.; Pashley, D. H. Evaluation of regional bond strength of resin cement to endodontic surfaces. *J. Endod.*, 2001, 27, 321– 4.

Gatewood, R. S. Endodontic materials. *Dent. Clin. North Am.*, 2007, 51, 695-712.

Gomes, B. P.; Berber, V. B.; Montagner, F.; Sena, N. T.; Zaia, A. A.; Ferraz, C. C.; Souza-Filho, F. J. Residual effects and surface alterations in disinfected gutta-percha and resilon cones. *J. Endod.*, 2007, 33, 948–51.

Gomes, B. P.; Vianna, M. E.; Matsumoto, C. U.; Rossi Vde, P.; Zaia, A. A.; Ferraz, C. C.; Souza Filho, F. J. Disinfection of gutta-percha cones with chlorhexidine and sodium hypochlorite. *Oral Surg. Oral Med. Oral Pathol. Oral Radiol. Endod.*, 2005, 100, 512–7.

Gomes, B. P.; Vianna, M. E.; Sena, N. T.; Zaia, A. A.; Ferraz, C. C.; Souza Filho, F. J. In vitro evaluation of the antimicrobial activity of calcium hydroxide combined with chlorhexidine gel used as intracanal medicament. *Oral Surg. Oral Med. Oral Pathol. Oral Radiol. Endod.*, 2006;102:544-50.

Gwinnett, A. J. Quantitative contribution of resin infiltration/hybridization to dentin bonding. *Am. J. Dent.*, 1993, 6, 7–9.

Hansen, S. E.; Swift, E. J. Microleakage with Gluma: effects of unfilled resin polymerization and storage time. *Am. J. Dent.*, 1989, 2, 266–8.

Hashem, A. A.; Ghoneim, A. G.; Lutfy, R. A.; Fouda, M. Y. The effect of different irrigating solutions on bond strength of two root canal-filling systems. *J. Endod.*, 2009, 35, 537-40.

Hebling, J.; Pashley, D. H.; Tjaderhane, L.; Tay, F. R. Chlorhexidine arrests subclinical degradation of dentin hybrid layers in vivo. *J. Dent. Res.*, 2005, 84, 741– 6.

Isci, S.; Yoldas, O.; Dumani, A. Effects of sodium hypochlorite and chlorhexidine solutions on Resilon (synthetic polymer based root canal filling material) cones: an atomic force microscopy study. *J. Endod.*, 2006, 32, 967–9.

Jacobovitz, M.; Vianna, M. E.; Pandolfelli, V. C.; Oliveira, I. R.; Rossetto, H. L.; Gomes, B. P. Root canal filling with cements based on mineral aggregates: an in vitro analysis of bacterial microleakage. *Oral Surg. Oral Med. Oral Pathol. Oral Radiol. Endod.*, 2009, 108, 140-4.

Jeansonne, M. J.; White, R. R. A comparison of 2.0% chlorhexidine gluconate and 5.25% sodium hypochlorite as antimicrobial endodontic irrigants. *J. Endod.*, 1994, 20, 276–8.

Kim, S. K.; Kim, Y. O. Influence of calcium hydroxide intracanal medication on apical seal. *Int. Endod. J.*, 2002, 35, 623– 8.

Kim, Y. K.; Grandini, S.; Ames, J. M.; Gu, L. S.; Kim, S. K.; Pashley, D. H.; Gutmann, J. L.; Tay, F. R. Critical review on methacrylate resin-based root canal sealers. *J. Endod.*, 2010, 36, 383-99.

Krishnamurthy, S. and Sudhakaran, S. Evaluation and prevention of the precipitate formed on interaction between sodium hypochlorite and chlorhexidine. *J. Endod.*, . 2010, 36, 1154-7.

Lai, S. C.; Mak, Y. F.; Cheung, G. S.; Osório, R.; Toledano, M.; Carvalho, R. M.; Tay, F. R.; Pashley, D. H. Reversal of compromised bonding to oxidized etched dentin. *J. Dent. Res.*, 2001, 80, 1919 –24.

Lambrianidis, T.; Margelos, J.; Beltes, P. Removal efficiency of calcium hydroxide dressing from the root canal. *J. Endod.*, 1999, 25, 85– 8.

Limkangwalmongkol, S.; Burscher, P.; Abbott, P. V., Sandler, A. B.; Bishop, B. M. A comparative study of the apical leakage of four root canal sealers and laterally condensed gutta percha. *J. Endod.*, 1991, 17, 495.

Mader, C.; Baumgartner, J. C.; Peters, D. D. Scanning electron microscopic investigation of the smeared layer on root canal walls. *J. Endod.*, 1984, 10, 477-83.

Mallmann, A.; Jacques, L. B.; Valandro, L. F.; Mathias, P.; Muench, A. Microtensile Bond strength of light- and self-cured adhesive systems to intraradicular dentin using a translucent fiber post. *Oper. Dent.*, 2005, 30, 500–6.

Mannocci, F.; Pilecki, P.; Bertelli, E.; Watson, T. F. Density of dentinal tubules affects the tensile strength of root dentin. *Dent. Mater.*, 2004, 20, 293– 6.

Mc Comb, D.; Smith, D. A preliminary scanning electron microscopic study of root canals after endodontic procedures. *J. Endod.*, 1975, 1, 238-42.

McDonnell, G.; Russell, A. Antiseptics and disinfectants: activity, action, and resistance. *Clin. Microbiol. Rev.*, 1999, 12, 147–79.

Meerbeek, B.; De Munck, J.; Yoshida, Y.; Inoue, S.; Vargas, M.; Vijay, P. Buonocore memorial lecture. Adhesion to enamel and dentin: current status and future challenges. *Oper. Dent.*, 2003, 28, 215–35.

Mjor, I. A.; Smith, M. R.; Ferrari, M.; Mannocci, F. The structure of dentine in the apical region of human teeth. *Int. Endod. J.*, 2001, 34, 346 –53.

Moreira, D. M.; Almeida, J. F.; Ferraz, C. C.; Gomes, B. P.; Line, S. R.; Zaia, A. A. Structural analysis of bovine root dentin after use of different endodontics auxiliary chemical substances. *J. Endod.*, 2009, 35, 1023-7.

Moreira, D. M.; de Andrade Feitosa, J. P.; Line, S. R.; Zaia, A. A. Effects of reducing agents on birefringence dentin collagen after use of different endodontic auxiliary chemical substances. *J. Endod.*, 2011, 37, 1406-11.

Morris, M. D.; Lee, K. W.; Agee, K. A.; Bouillaguet, S.; Pashley, D. H. Effects of sodium hypochlorite and RC-prep on bond strengths of resin cement to endodontic surfaces. *J. Endod.*, 2001, 27, 753–7.

Muniz, L.; Mathias, P. The influence of sodium hypochlorite and root canal sealers on post retention in different dentin regions. *Oper. Dent.*, 2005, 30, 533–9.

Naenni, N.; Thoma, K.; Zehnder, M. Soft tissue dissolution capacity of currently used and potential endodontic irrigants. *J. Endod.*, 2004, 30, 785–7.

Nair, P. N. R.; Sjögreen, U.; Key, G.; Kahnberg, K. E.; Sundqvist, G. Intraradicular bacteria and fungi in root-filled, asymptomatic human teeth with therapy- resistant periapical lesions: A longterm light and electron microscopic follow-up study. *J. Endod.*, 1990, 16, 580-8.

Nakabayashi, N.; Kojima, K.; Masuhara, E. The promotion of adhesion by the infiltration of monomers into tooth substrates. *J. Biomed. Mater. Res.*, 1982, 16, 265–9.

Nakashima, K.; Terata, R. Effect of pH modified EDTA solution to the properties of dentin. *J. Endod.*, 2005, 31, 47-9.

Neelakantan, P.; Subbarao, C.; Subbarao, C. V.; De-Deus, G.; Zehnder, M. The impact of root dentinee conditioning on sealing ability and push-out Bond strength of na epoxy resin root canal sealer. *Int. Endod. J.,* 2011, 44, 491–8.

Nikaido, T.; Takano, Y.; Sasafuchi, Y.; Burrow, M. F.; Tagami, J. Bond strengths to endodontically- treated teeth. *Am. J. Dent.,* 1999, 12, 177– 80.

Okino, L. A.; Siqueira, E. L.; Santos, M.; Bombana, A. C.; Figueiredo, J. A. Dissolution of pulp tissue by aqueous solution of chlorhexidine digluconate and chlorhexidine digluconate gel. *Int. Endod. J.,* 2004, 37, 38-41.

Ozturk, B.; Özer, F. Effect of NaOCl on bond strengths of bonding agents to pulp chamber lateral walls. *J. Endod.,* 2004, 30, 362–5.

Perdigão, J.; Lopes, M.; Geraldeli, S.; Lopes, G. C.; Garcia-Godoy, F. Effect of a sodium hypochlorite gel on dentin bonding. *Dent. Mater.,* 2000, 16, 311–23.

Pereira, P. N.; Okuda, M.; Sano, H.; Yoshikawa, T.; Burrow, M. F.; Tagami, J. Effect of intrinsic wetness and regional difference on dentin bond strength. *Dent. Mater.,* 1999, 15, 46 –53.

Prado, M.; De Assis, D. F.; Gomes, B. P.; Simão, R. A. Effect of disinfectant solutions on the surface free energy and wettability of filling material. *J. Endod.,* 2011, 37, 980-2.

Prado, M.; Gusman, H.; Gomes, B. P.; Simão, R.A. Effect of disinfectant solutions on gutta-percha and resilon cones. *Microsc. Res. Tech.,* 2012, 75, 791-5.

Prado, M.; Gusman, H.; Gomes, B. P.; Simão, R. A. Scanning electron microscopic investigation of the effectiveness of phosphoric acid in smear layer removal when compared with EDTA and citric acid. *J. Endod.* 2011, 37, 255-8.

Prado, M.; Gusman, H.; Gomes, B. P.; Simão, R. A. The importance of final rinse after disinfection of gutta-percha and Resilon cones. *Oral Surg. Oral Med. Oral Pathol. Oral Radiol. Endod.,* 2011, 111, e21-4.

Prado, M.; Gusman, H.; Gomes, B. P. F. A.; Simão, R. A. A Comparative Study of the Smear Layer Removal Using Scanning Electronic Microscopy and Atomic Force Microscopy. *Adv. Microsc. Res.,* 2012, 7, 21-25.

Prasansuttiporn, T.; Nakajima, M.; Kunawarote, S.; Foxton, R.M.; Tagami, J. Effect of reducing agents on bond strength to NaOCl-treated dentin. *Dent. Mater.,* 2011, 27, 229-34.

Ramé-hart Instrument Co. Information on Contact Angle. 26th Aug. 2012. Available from: URL: http://www.ramehart.com/contactangle.htm

Royal, M. J.; Willianson, A. E.; Drake, D. R. Comparison of 5.25% sodium hypochlorite, MTAD and 2% chlorhexidine in the rapid disinfection of prolycaprolactane-based root canal filling materials. *J. Endod.*, 2007, 33, 42–4.

Russell, P.; Batchelor, D.; Thornton, J. SEM and AFM: Complementary Techniques for High Resolution Surface Investigations. (15th july 2012). Available from: URL: http://personal.cityu.edu.hk/~appkchu/AP5301/ SEM%20and%20AFM%20-%20Complementary%20techniques.pdf

Schwartz, R. S. Adhesive dentistry and endodontics. Part 2: bonding in the root canal system-the promise and the problems: a review. *J. Endod.*, 2006, 32, 1125-34.

Sevimay, S.; Oztan, M. D.; Dalat, D. Effects of calcium hydroxide paste medication on coronal leakage. *J. Oral Rehabil.*, 2004, 31, 240–4.

Shokouhinejad, N.; Sharifian, M. R.; Aligholi, M.; Assadian, H.; Tabor, R. K.; Nekoofar, M. H. The sealing ability of resilon and gutta-parcha following different smear layer removal methods: an ex vivo study. *Oral. Surg. Oral Med. Oral Pathol. Oral Radiol. Endod.*, 2010, 110, e45-9.

Short, R. D.; Dorn, S. O.; Kuttler, S. The crystallization of sodium hypochlorite on gutta-percha cones after the rapid-sterilization technique: an SEM study. *J. Endod.*, 2003, 29, 670-3.

Spangberg, L. Biological effects of root canal filling materials. IV. Effect in vitro of solubilized root canal filling materials on HeLa cells. *Odontol. Revy* 1969, 20, 289.

Tagami, J.; Tao, L.; Pashley, D. H. Correlation among dentin depth, permeability, and bond strength of adhesive resin. *Dent. Mater.*, 1990, 6, 45–50.

Tao, L.; Pashley, D. H. Shear bond strengths to dentin: effects of surface treatments, depth and position. *Dent. Mater.*, 1988, 4, 371– 8.

Tay, F. R.; Hiraishi, N.; Pashley, D. H.; Loushine, R. J.; Weller, R. N.; Gillespie, W. T.; Doyle, M. D. Bondability of Resilon to a methacrylate-based root canal sealer. *J. Endod.*, 2006, 32, 133-7.

Tay, F. R.; Loushine, R. J.; Monticelli, F.; Weller, R. N.; Breschi, L.; Ferrari, M.; Pashley, D. H. Effectiveness of resin-coated gutta-percha cones and a dual-cured, hydrophilic methacrylate resin-based sealer in obturating root canals. *J. Endod.*, 2005, 31, 659-64.

Torabinejad, M.; Handysides, R.; Khademi, A. A.; Bakland, L. K. Clinical implications of the smear layer in endodontics: a review. *Oral Surg. Oral Med. Oral Pathol. Oral Radiol. Endod.,* 2002, 94, 658-66.

Valois, C. R.; Silva, L. P.; Azevedo, R. B. Structural effects of sodium hypochlorite solutions on gutta-percha cones: atomic force microscopy study. *J. Endod.,* 2005, 31, 749–51.

Valois, C. R.; Silva, L. P.; Azevedo, R. B.; Costa Jr, E. D. Atomic force microscopy study of gutta-percha cone topography. *Oral Surg. Oral Med. Oral Pathol. Oral Radiol. Endod.,* 2004, 98, 250-5.

Vilalta-Clemente, A.; Gloystein, K. Principles of Atomic Force Microscopy (AFM). *Physics of Advanced Materials Winter School,* 2008, 1-10

Vivacqua-Gomes, N.; Ferraz, C. C.; Gomes, B. P.; Zaia, A. A.; Teixeira, F. B.; Souza-Filho, F. J. Influence of irrigants on the coronal microleakage of laterally condensed gutta-percha root fillings. *Int. Endod. J.,* 2002, 35, 791-5.

Voutou, B.; Stefanaki E. Electron Microscopy: The Basics. *Physics of Advanced Materials Winter School,* 2008, 1-11.

Wennberg, A.; Ørstavik, D. Adhesion of root canal sealers to bovine dentin and gutta percha. *Int. Endod. J.,* 1990, 23, 13-9.

White, R. R.; Hays, G. L.; Janer, L.R. Residual antimicrobial activity after canal irrigation with chlorhexidine. *J. Endod.,* 1997, 23, 229–31.

Yesilsoy, C.; Whitaker, E.; Cleveland, D.; Phillips, E.; Trope, M. Antimicrobial and toxic effects of established and potential root canal irrigants. *J. Endod.,* 1995, 21, 513–5.

Yilmaz, Z.; Basbag, B.; Buzoglu, H. D.; Gümüsderelioglu, M. Effect of low-surface-tension EDTA solutions on the wettability of root canal dentin. *Oral Surg. Oral Med. Oral Pathol. Oral Radiol. Endod.,* 2011, 111, 109-14.

Yiu, C. K.; Garcia-Godoy, F.; Tay, F. R. A nanoleakage perspective on bonding to oxidized dentin. *J. Dent. Res.,* 2002, 81, 628 –32.

Yoshikawa, T.; Sano, H.; Burrow, M. F.; Tagami, J.; Pashley, D. H. Effects of dentin depth and cavity configuration on bond strength. *J. Dent Res.,* 1999, 78, 898 –905.

Yoshiyama, M.; Carvalho, R. M.; Sano, H.; Horner, J. A.; Brewer, P. D.; Pashley, D.H. Regional bond strengths of resins to human root dentine. *J. Dent.,* 1996, 24, 435– 42.

Yoshiyama, M.; Matsuo, T.; Ebisu, S.; Pashley, D. Regional bond strengths of self-etching/ self-priming adhesive systems. *J. Dent.,* 1998, 26, 609 –16.

Zehnder, M. Root canal irrigants. *J. Endod.,* 2006, 32, 389–98.

In: Recent Advances in Adhesions Research   ISBN: 978-1-62417-447-6
Editors: A. McFarland and M. Akins   © 2013 Nova Science Publishers, Inc.

Chapter 2

POLYSIALYLATED-NEURAL CELL ADHESION MOLECULE (PSA-NCAM) IN THE HUMAN NERVOUS SYSTEM AT PRENATAL, POSTNATAL AND ADULT AGES

Marina Quartu,[1]* Maria Pina Serra,[1] Marianna Boi,[1]
Roberto Demontis,[2] Tiziana Melis,[1] Laura Poddighe,[1]
Cristina Picci[1] and Marina Del Fiacco[1]
[1]Department of Biomedical Sciences, section of
Cytomorphology, University of Cagliari, Cittadella
Universitaria di Monserrato, Monserrato (Cagliari), Italy
[2]Department of Public Health, Clinical and Molecular Medicine,
Azienda Ospedaliero Universitaria, University of Cagliari,
Monserrato (Cagliari), Italy

ABSTRACT

The polysialylated form of the neural cell adhesion molecule (PSA-NCAM) has received much attention in recent years and it is often used

* Corresponding author: Marina Quartu. E-mail: quartu@unica.it. E-mail addresses: MPS: mpserra@unica.it. MB: marianna.boi@unica.it. TM: tiziana.melis@unica.it. DR: robertodemontis@medicina.unica.it. LP: laura.poddighe@unica.it. CP: picci@unica.it. MDF: dfiacco@unica.it.

as a marker of neuronal cells undergoing structural and functional changes. The association of NCAM with chains of polysialic acid is finely tuned throughout nervous system development to confer the molecule a role as negative modulator of cell adhesive properties thereby allowing neurons to undergo plastic changes, such as neurite outgrowth and synaptic reorganization, in both embryonic and adult life.

In adult mammals, PSA-NCAM expression persists in cerebral regions such as the hippocampus, the olfactory cortex, the medial prefrontal cortex, the amygdala, the hypothalamus, and terminal regions of primary sensory afferents where continuous remodelling has been described. In man, selected populations of central and peripheral neurons have been reported to express PSA-NCAM in normal conditions, supporting the concept of an involvement of this molecule in structural and functional plasticity throughout life. Accordingly, expression of PSA-NCAM is regulated in response to events involving synaptic structural plasticity such as learning, memory consolidation, chronic stress or chronic antidepressant treatment and different types of neuronal lesion models. Interestingly, its localization in subpopulations of primary sensory neurons suggests that PSA-NCAM may also have a part in the processing of somatosensory information. Here, by presenting both original observations from our laboratory and literature data, we review knowledge on the occurrence of the molecule in sensory ganglia, brainstem nuclei and hippocampal formation of the human nervous system at different developmental ages spanning from prenatal and postnatal to adult life. As morphological support of the possible interactions of PSA-NCAM with neurotrophic factors, data on PSA-NCAM codistribution with the neurotrophin BDNF in the brainstem are reviewed and novel findings on PSA-NCAM/BDNF codistribution and colocalization in the hippocampus are presented.

INTRODUCTION

The polysialylated form of the cell surface glycoprotein neural cell adhesion molecule (PSA-NCAM) is a dynamically regulated post-translational modification of NCAM (Rutishauser et al., 1996; Rutishauser, 2008). Due to its large excluded volume, PSA can produce sufficient physical hindrance between apposing membranes to attenuate intercellular adhesion (Rutishauser, 2008; Johnson et al., 2005).

The highest expression of PSA-NCAM occurs in the developing nervous system, where it is generally considered a promoter of neural plasticity, allowing migration of neural and nonneural precursors and facilitating axonal pathfinding and synaptogenesis (Kiss et al., 1997; El Maarouf et al., 2003). In the normal adult brain of experimental animals NCAM generally displays low levels of polysialylation (Angata et al., 2003), with the exception of limited areas such as the hippocampus, the hypothalamus, the olfactory cortex and terminal regions of primary sensory afferents, which are believed to maintain a capability for morphological reorganization throughout life (Seki et al., 1993a; Kajikawa et al., 1997; Theodosis et al., 1999; El Maarouf et al., 2005; Luzzati et al., 2009).

The PSA-NCAM levels and distribution have been shown to increase in learning and memory (Becker et al., 1996; Fox et al., 2000; Ronn et al., 2000), chronic stress conditions (Pham et al., 20033; Sandy et al., 2003; Nacher et al., 2004) and several lesion models such as ischemia, epilepsy, brain trauma, and transected/crushed peripheral nerves (Rutishauser, 2008; Bonfanti et al., 1996; Bonfanti, 2006; Iwai et al., 2001; Emery et al., 2003; Singh et al., 2005; Franz et al., 2005).

Interestingly, the potential of PSA-NCAM expressing endogenous cells in promoting brain tissue repair (Nguyen et al., 2003; El Maarouf et al., 2006; 2008) and a role for this molecule in neuroprotection (Duveau et al., 2007) have been pointed out.

An alternative role of PSA-NCAM has been related to increasing the concentration of soluble factors, such as neurotrophic factors, in the vicinity of cell membranes (reviewed in Bonfanti, 2006). In fact, PSA-NCAM has been shown to facilitate the interaction of BDNF with trkB (Muller et al., 2000; Vutskits et al., 2001) and to regulate the expression of the p75 neurotrophin receptor (Gascon et al., 2007), thereby modulating the neuronal sensitivity to trophic factors.

Studies on expression in the human nervous system lay the ground for understanding the potentiality of neural cells for dynamic changes and plasticity in response to environmental cues. So far, data regarding the occurrence of the molecule in the normal human nervous system have shown the localization of PSA-NCAM in discrete regions of the early fetal forebrain and suggest its role in developmental processes, such as neuronal migration and transitory axonal projections (Ulfig et al., 2004), and onset of myelination (Jakovcevski et al., 2007).

We have reported the occurrence of PSA-NCAM later in development in the trigeminal ganglion and nucleus and in brainstem precerebellar nuclei of pre- and full-term newborns, territories where its expression is maintained throughout life (Quartu et al., 2008; 2010).

Table 1. List of specimens

Case	Age	Sex	Cause of death	Post-mortem delay	Method	Specimen
1	21 w.g.	M	Cardio-respiratory failure	35 h	WB, IHC	Hippocampus
2	28 w.g	F	Cardio-respiratory failure	34 h	WB	Medulla oblongata
3	28 w.g	F	Cardio-respiratory failure	37 h	IHC	Brainstem, TG
4	34 w.g.	F	Cardio-respiratory failure	34 h	WB	Medulla oblongata
5	35 w.g.	M	Cardio-respiratory failure	25 h	IHC	Hippocampus
6	36 w.g.	F	Cardio-respiratory failure	26 h	IHC	Brainstem, TG, hippocampus
7	40 w.g.	M	Cardio-respiratory failure	37 h	WB	Hippocampus
8	7 d	F	Pneumonitis	44	IHC	Hippocampus
9	8 m	M	Broncopneumonitis	45 h	IHC	Medulla oblongata, mesencephalon
10	42 y	M	Cardio-respiratory failure	37 h	IHC	Brainstem, TG
11	47 y	F	Pneumonitis	50 h	WB, IHC	Hippocampus, brainstem, TG
12	50 y	F	Embolysm of pulmonary artery	26 h	WB	Hippocampus
13	51 y	F	Myocardial infarction	54 h	WB, IHC	Hippocampus, brainstem
14	52 y	M	Cardio-respiratory failure	45 h	IHC	Medulla oblongata, mesencephalon
15	55 y	F	Cardio-respiratory failure	28 h	IHC	Hippocampus
16	60 y	F	Myocardial infarction	45 h	WB	Medulla oblongata, mesencephalon
17	67 y	F	Thromboembolysm of pulmonary artery	38 h	IHC	Brainstem
18	69 y	M	Myocardial infarction	45 h	WB	Medulla oblongata, mesencephalon
19	71 a	M	Myocardial infarction	30 h	IHC	Hippocampus
20	75 a	M	Embolysm of pulmonary artery	30 h	IHC	Hippocampus
21	81 y	M	Ruptured abdominal aortic aneurysm	39 h	WB	Medulla oblongata
22	82 y	F	Myocardial infarction	28 h	WB	Hippocampus
23	88 y	M	Embolysm of pulmonary artery	47 h	WB, IHC	Hippocampus, brainstem, TG

Legend: F, female; h, hours; IHC, immunohistochemistry; M, male; m, months; TG, trigeminal ganglion; w.g., weeks of gestation; WB, western blot.

The persistence of PSA-NCAM has been further shown in cerebral cortex (Ní Dhúill et al., 1999; Arellano et al., 2002; Varea et al., 2007), amydgala (Varea et al., 2012) and peripheral nerve (Roche et al., 1997), where altered expression of the molecule has also been described in a number of neuropathological conditions (Roche et al., 1997; Barbeau et al., 1995; Mikkonen et al., 1998; 1999; Mathern et al., 2002; Charles et al., 2002; Weber et al., 2006).

Such studies certainly represent the ground work for future analyses of pathological tissue specimens and, hopefully, for prospective applications in neuronal protection and repair.

In this chapter, by presenting both original observations from our laboratory and literature data, we review knowledge on the immunohistochemical occurrence of the molecule in the trigeminal sensory ganglion, in the morphofunctional heterogenous neuronal populations of the brainstem and in the hippocampal formation of the human nervous system at different developmental ages spanning from prenatal and postnatal to adult life.

Furthermore, in order to investigate the issue of possible interactions of PSA-NCAM with neurotrophic factors, we review data on PSA-NCAM/BDNF codistribution in several areas of the brainstem (Quartu et al., 2010) and report novel observations on PSA-NCAM/BDNF codistribution and colocalization in the hippocampus. A list of examined human specimens is reported in Table I.

RESULTS

PSA-NCAM Tissue Localization

Western Blot

In tissue homogenates of human medulla oblongata and hippocampus, at all examined ages, the anti-PSA-NCAM antibody (MAB5324, Chemicon, US) labelled a single broad band (Figures 1A, 2A) at a level corresponding to the expected molecular weight (Dubois et al., 1994; Quartu et al., 2008; 2010). By contrast, and in agreement with immunohistochemical observations (below), no stained bands were detected in samples of human mesencephalic tissue (Figure 1A, lane 4). Control immunostaining carried out with the anti-PSA-NCAM antibody preabsorbed with 5mg of colominic acid (alfa-2-8-linked sialic polymer colominic acid) resulted in no staining (Figure 1B).

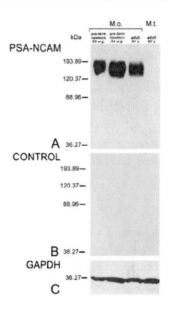

Figure 1. Western blot analysis of PSA-NCAM and GAPDH in human brainstem homogenates of human pre-term newborn (cases 2, 4) (first and second lane, respectively) and adult medulla oblongata (M.o.) (case 21) (third lane), and adult mesencephalic tegmentum (M.t.) (case 18) (fourth lane). CONTROL: representative control immunostaining. h, hours of post-mortem interval; w.g., weeks of gestation; y, years.

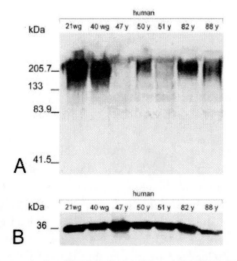

Figure 2. Western blot analysis of PSA-NCAM (A) and GAPDH (B) in human hippocampal tissue homogenates (cases 1, 7, 11, 12, 21, 22, 23). wg, weeks of gestation; y, years.

The thickness and staining intensity of the bands were generally more pronounced in pre- and full-term newborn versus adult tissue (Figure 2A). In the case of hippocampus, of which several specimens were examined, a high degree of individual variability among the adult specimens was obvious (Figure 2).

Immunohistochemistry

The vast majority of PSA-NCAM-immunolabelled structures appeared as neuronal cell bodies and processes showing mainly a peripheral immunoreactivity suggestive of membrane labelling and as varicose and smooth filaments and punctate elements, interpreted as nerve fibres and terminals, often with a plexiform aspect.

Trigeminal ganglion. PSA-NCAM-like immunoreactivity (LI) was localized to neuronal perikarya, nerve fibres in bundles and in isolated profiles between neurons, and to satellite and Schwann cells; further, intense cytoplasmic staining and networks of positive pericellular fibres occurred in adult tissue whereas in the newborn they were detectable only occasionally (Figure 3).

At fetal age, a number of neuronal cell bodies were surrounded by immunoreactive material, which may be interpreted as membrane labelling, though aspects reminiscent of labelled satellite cells could be found; rare neurons showed a cytoplasmic staining (Figure 3A).

In adult tissue, several neurons showed a peripheral immunoreactivity suggestive of membrane labelling (Figure 3C, D). However, a number of them seemed surrounded by immunostained satellite cells (Figure 3 D, E), which made it difficult to unequivocally identify a membrane staining and to ascertain a neuronal labelling.

On the other hand, a number of perikarya also showed cytoplasmic labelling, thus allowing a morphometric analysis. This was done considering only the cell sections where both staining of the cytoplasmic compartment and the nucleus were clearly detectable (Figure 3B, C). In the TG specimen from an adult subject, such cells amounted to about $6.4 \pm 0.075\%$ of the total ganglionic population.

About 70% of labelled neurons have a mean cell diameter ranging from 22 μm to 34 μm, thus falling in the class of small- and medium-sized cells, whereas the remaining of them fell in the large size range. Varicose fibres could be found either isolated or as bundles of variable density (Figure 3C-E). A few non immunolabelled neuronal cell bodies appeared surrounded by immunoreactive varicose nerve fibres (Figure 3E, F).

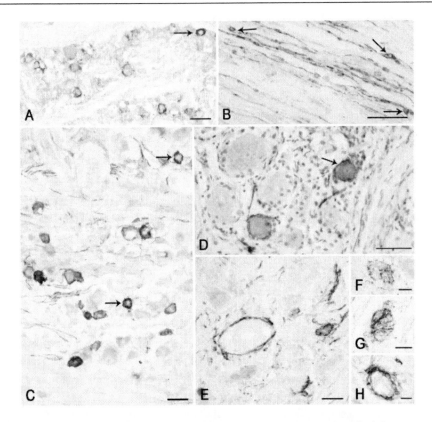

Figure 3. PSA-NCAM in the human pre-term newborn (A,B: case 6) and adult trigeminal ganglion (C-H: case 10, C-F: case 22). A-E: immunostained perikarya and nerve fibres; B: immunoreactive nerve fibres; arrows point to immunostained Schwann cells; in D, a tissue section immunostained for PSA-NCAM and co-stained with modified Mayer's hematoxylin is shown. Arrows in C and D point to PSA-NCAM immunostained neurons whose nucleus is clearly detectable. E, H: the immunolabelling appears localized to the satellite cells surrounding non immunoreactive neurons. F, G: pericellular varicose arborisations around non immunoreactive neurons. Scale bars: A-E = 50 μm; F = 25 μm; G, H = 20 μm.

Brainstem. PSA-NCAM-LI was mainly distributed at the level of the medulla oblongata and pons and was scarce in the mesencephalon. The distribution pattern was uneven and remained fairly constant in specimens of different age, though changes in the density of immunoreactive structures and in the staining intensity may occur in newborn compared to adult specimens, e.g. as in the spinal trigeminal nucleus, caudal part (Figure 4). Immunoreactivity also occurred in discretely localized glial structures, such as the dorsal median septum and the ependymal lining.

At caudal level of the medulla oblongata, the spinal trigeminal nucleus harbored the bulk of immunoreactivity. The trigeminal sensory nuclear complex showed an uneven distribution of immunoreactive elements.

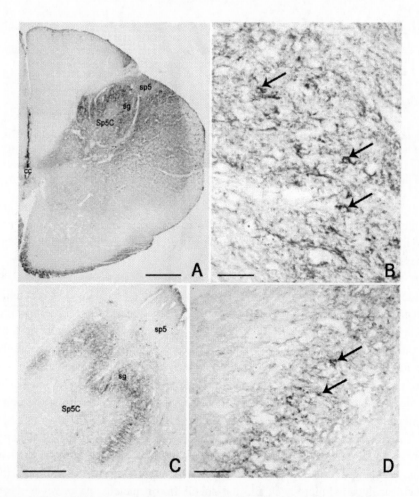

Figure 4. PSA-NCAM in the human pre-term (A, B: case 6) and adult medulla oblongata, caudal level (case 23) (C, D). A: panoramic view of the right half of a section at the boundary with the spinal cord. B: higher magnification of the substantia gelatinosa (sg) of the spinal trigeminal nucleus, caudal part (Sp5C); arrows point to labelled neuronal perikarya. C: a panoramic view of the right side spinal trigeminal nucleus, caudal part (Sp5C) , at the boundary with the spinal cord. D: higher magnification of the substantia gelatinosa; arrows point to labelled neurons in the spinal nucleus substantia gelatinosa (sg). sp5, spinal trigeminal tract; cc, central canal; sp5, spinal trigeminal tract. Scale bars: A, C = 500 μm; B = 50 μm; D = 100 μm.

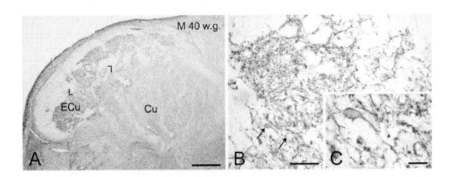

Figure 5. PSA-NCAM in the human full-term (case 7) external cuneate nucleus (ECu), left side. B: higher magnification of the area framed in A; C, higher magnification of the cell bodies pointed by arrows in B. Cu, cuneate nucleus. Scale bars: A, 500 µm; B, 50 µm; C, 20 µm.

At all ages examined, PSA-NCAM-LI was restricted to the spinal trigeminal nucleus (Figures 4; 6), where it was represented by neuronal cell bodies and processes, and was virtually absent in the principal and mesencephalic nuclei.

At fetal age, immunoreactive fibres were present in the spinal tract of the trigeminal nerve (Figures 4A; 6A) and in the spinal nucleus pars caudalis, where a rich plexus and neuronal cell bodies occurred in the substantia gelatinosa (Figure 4A,B), and in the pars interpolaris (Figure 6A). In adult tissue, the immunostaining persisted in the substantia gelatinosa whereas the spinal tract and the magnocellular subnucleus harbored rare elements (Figure 4C, D). More rostrally, the tegmentum showed several areas of intense to moderate immunoreactivity including sensory and motor cranial nerve nuclei, reticular formation and precerebellar nuclei (Figures 5-7).

At all ages examined, neuronal perikarya and plexuses of labelled nerve fibres could be observed in the commissural nucleus and solitary nuclear complex (Figures 6A; 7A,B), the vestibular system (Figures 6A; 7C, D), the cochlear nuclei (Figure 6A), and the dorsal motor nucleus of the vagus nerve (Figures 6A; 7F). While PSA-NCAM-LI was scarce in the newborn (Figure 6A), in the adult the hypoglossal nucleus showed a moderate immunostaining comprising nerve fibre plexuses surrounding non immunoreactive neuronal cell bodies (Figure 7E).

Immunoreactive fibre networks and terminals, and peripherally labelled neurons, were also present in the gracile nucleus, external cuneate nucleus (Figure 5), perihypoglossal nuclei (Figure 6), inferior olive complex (Figure 6), arcuate nucleus and reticular formation nuclei (Figures 6A; 7G).

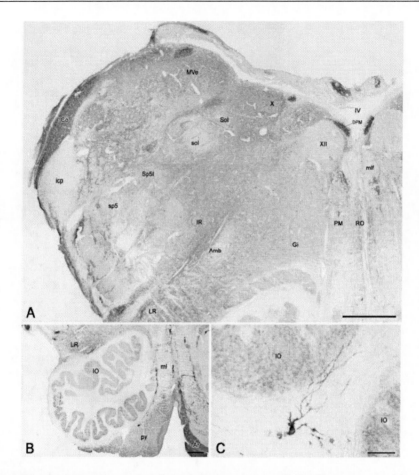

Figure 6. PSA-NCAM in the human pre-term newborn medulla oblongata, rostral level (case 6). A: panoramic view of the left side dorsal quadrant at the level of the rostral hypoglossal nucleus cell column. B: left side ventral quadrant showing immunolabelling in the lateral reticular nucleus (LR), inferior olive (IO), pyramidal tract (py), and arcuate nucleus (Ar). C: a positive cell in the white matter around the inferior olive, which extends long labelled processes towards the nucleus. Ar, arcuate nucleus; Co, dorsal cochlear nucleus; DPM, dorsal paramedian nucleus; Gi, gigantocellular nucleus; icp, inferior cerebellar peduncle; IO, inferior olive; IPo, interpositus hypoglossi nucleus; IR, intermediate reticular nucleus; LR, lateral reticular nucleus; ml, medial lemniscus; mlf, medial longitudinal fasciculus; mlf, medial longitudinal fasciculus; MVe, medial vestibular nucleus; PM, paramedian reticular nucleus; py, pyramidal tract; RO, raphe obscurus nucleus; Sol, solitary nucleus; sol, solitary tract; sp5, spinal trigeminal tract; Sp5I, spinal trigeminal nucleus, interpolar part; IV, fourth ventricle; X, dorsal motor nucleus of the vagus nerve; XII, hypoglossal nucleus. Scale bars: A, B = 500 μm; C = 20 μm.

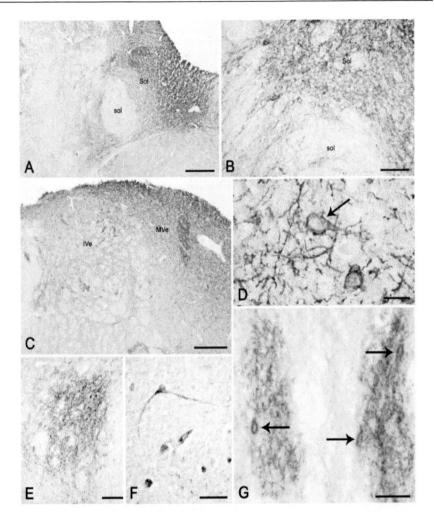

Figure 7. PSA-NCAM in the human adult medulla oblongata (case 10). A, B: left side solitary nucleus (Sol) and tract (sol). C: left side inferior (IVe) and medial vestibular (MVe) nuclei. D: a neuronal perikaryon with membrane labelling (arrow) and fibres in the neuropil of the medial vestibular nucleus. E: hypoglossal nucleus. F: dorsal motor nucleus of the vagus nerve. G: perikarya with membrane labelling (arrows) and fibre networks in the raphe obscurus nucleus. Scale bars: A, C, E = 500 μm; B = 100 μm; D = 20 μm; F, G = 50 μm.

In the principal, dorsal and medial accessory, and conterminal nucleus of the inferior olive PSA-NCAM-LI labelled mainly the neuropil (Figure 6B, C). Though the immunostaining of these nuclei occurred in young and adult specimens, the distribution pattern and quality of PSA-NCAM-LI varied among specimens of different age.

In the 21weeks of gestation (w.g.) pre-term newborn, the grey matter had a sandwich-like aspect, with two bands of immunostaining flanking a central lighter zone. In the 35 w.g. pre-term newborn and successive ages (Figure 6B), the neuropil was homogeneously immunoreactive and contained membrane-labelled cell bodies.

At all ages examined, the white matter surrounding the olivary nuclei harbored isolated positive cell bodies intensely stained for PSA-NCAM, which extend long processes towards the nucleus (Figure 6C).

In the reticular formation, positive fibre networks and peripherally labelled neurons were located in the paramedian reticular (Figure 6A), raphe obscurus (Figures 6A; 7G), gigantocellular (Figure 6A), central reticular, intermediate reticular and lateral reticular nuclei (Figure 6A). The arcuate nucleus also contained a very thick plexus of PSA-NCAM-positive nerve fibres and scattered cell bodies (Figure 6B).

In newborn specimens, the pyramidal tract was moderately stained (Figure 6B); nerve fibres, isolated or grouped in small bundlets, occurred across the medial lemniscus (Figure 6B), in the course of the vestibular nerve and, at early prenatal age, in the white matter between the vestibular nuclei and the cerebellum.

In the pons, bundles of strongly immunoreactive nerve fibres ran in the eighth cranial nerve and reached the pontine territory of the vestibular and cochlear nuclei, which harbored immunoreactive cell bodies. In the newborn, at caudalmost levels, the oral part of the dorsal paramedian nucleus showed an intense immunoreactivity due to positive neuronal perikarya and processes. The subependymal grey contained a light punctate labelling throughout. In the adult, a diffuse weak staining was also appreciable in the locus coeruleus neuropil in between the unstained pigmented neurons. The caudal pontine, gigantocellular, parvocellular, reticulotegmental, and oral pontine reticular nuclei contained sparse neuronal cell bodies with peripheral membrane labelling and rare punctate and filamentous elements. The pontine nuclei showed an intense labelling due to peripherally stained neuronal perikarya and a meshwork of thin filamentous and punctate elements in between them. Labelled nerve fibres, isolated or in bundles, occurred across the medial longitudinal fasciculus, medial lemniscus and lateral lemniscus.

In the quadrigeminal plate, sparse neuronal perikarya occurred in the external and pericentral nuclei of the inferior colliculus, the intercollicular region and the superior colliculus. A diffuse immunostaining, occasionally localized to neuronal perikarya, occurred in the periaqueductal grey and in the territory of the median and dorsal raphe nuclei. PSA-NCAM-LI in the red nucleus, virtually absent at prenatal and adult age, revealed a delicate meshwork of positive nerve fibres in the full-term newborn. A diffuse immunostaining could be observed in the substantia nigra only in adult tissue. The cerebral peduncle harbored transversely sectioned labelled fibres. Close to the ventral surface of the caudal mesencephalon, positive nerve fibres formed a small area of dense immunoreactivity located along the ventromedial boundary of the crus cerebri.

Hippocampus. At all examined ages, PSA-NCAM-LI was distributed throughout the hippocampus and labelled rare neuronal cell bodies, nerve fibres and terminals (Figures 8; 9; 11; 12).

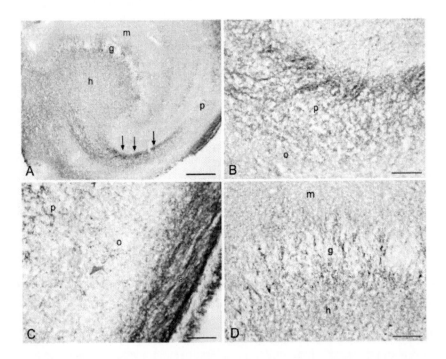

Figure 8. PSA-NCAM in the human newborn hippocampus (case 8). A: panoramic view of the Ammon's horn and fascia dentata; arrows point to nerve fibers in proximity and within the pyramidal layer of the CA3 sector; B: pyramidal layer of the CA3 sector; C: nerve fibers in the pyramidal layer of the CA1 sector and in the alveus; D: fibers and punctate elements in the fascia dentata. a, alveus; g, granule cell layer; h, hilus; m, molecular layer; p, pyramidal layer; o, stratum oriens. Scale bars: A = 500 μm; B, C = 100 μm; D = 20 μm.

In pre- and full term newborns, immunoreactive elements appeared diffusely distributed in the neuropil of both Ammon's horn and the fascia dentata (Figure 8). Labelled granular cells were generally rare. The inner part of the molecular layer showed a light punctate immunostaining in the pre-term newborns (Figure 8A), whereas it appeared devoid of PSA-NCAM-LI in the full-term newborn. Nerve fibre systems were particularly dense in the CA3 sector of Ammon's horn, where their course resembled that of the mossy fibers, and in the alveus (Figure 8A).

Compared to newborn specimens, in the adult the labelling acquires a more definite localization (Figure 9). Positive structures were represented by nerve fibres and a number of immunostained neurons, often of multipolar aspect, distributed in the pyramidal layer (Figure 9A, B) and stratum oriens of Ammon's horn. Numerous neuronal processes occupied the stratum radiatum (Figure 9A) whereas the stratum lacunosum moleculare appeared almost devoid of immunoreactivity (Figure 9A).

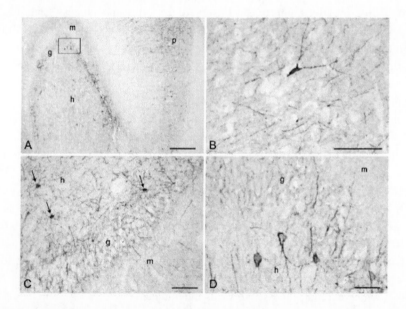

Figure 9. PSA-NCAM in the human adult hippocampus (case 19). A: panoramic view of the Ammon's horn and fascia dentata; B: positive neuron in the pyramidal layer of the CA1 sector; C: higher magnification of the microscopic field squared in A; nerve fibers in the hilus and granule cell layer of the fascia dentata; arrows point to positive hilar neurons; D: multipolar neurons in the hilus of the fascia dentata. g, granule cell layer; h, hilus; m, molecular layer; p, pyramidal layer. Scale bars: A = 500 μm; B, C = 100 μm; D = 20 μm.

In the fascia dentata, the hilus and granular layer contained rare positive neurons; a higher number of small positive neurons, showing mainly a peripheral staining in their soma and proximal dendritic processes, occurred in the infragranular layer (Figure 9A, C, D). A fine network of nerve fibers occurred around the non immunoreactive granular cells (Figure 9C). A very light dust-like immunostaining was present in the neuropil of the outer part of the molecular layer (Figure 9A, C).

PSA-NCAM/BDNF CODISTRIBUTION

Brainstem. Analysis of adjacent sections immunostained for PSA-NCAM and BDNF revealed codistribution in several brainstem nuclei (Figure 10). In neuronal perikarya, PSA-NCAM-LI appeared mostly as peripheral staining, whereas BDNF-LI appeared as intracytoplasmic granules. Immunoreactive nerve fibres and terminals were observed for both substances. Like PSA-NCAM, the distribution pattern of BDNF-LI was uneven and, with little exceptions, remained rather steady among the different ages examined.

In the medulla oblongata, both PSA-NCAM- and BDNF-LI occurred in the external cuneate nucleus, perihypoglossal nuclei, inferior olive complex, arcuate nucleus and lateral reticular formation.

In the perihypoglossal nuclei, such as the interfascicular nucleus (Figure 10A, B), PSA-NCAM-LI labelled both neurons and thick fibre networks while BDNF immunostaining occurred mainly in neuronal cell bodies. The inferior olive subnuclei showed mainly a neuropil immunostaining for PSA-NCAM (Figure 10C), whereas BDNF-LI was present in a number of neurons (Figure 10D).

The immunoreactivity for both substances was particularly rich in the conterminal nucleus (Figure 10C, D). Interestingly, at all ages examined, and similarly to PSA-NCAM (see Figure 6), the white matter surrounding the olivary nuclei harbored isolated positive cell bodies intensely stained for BDNF, which extend processes towards the nucleus.

The arcuate nucleus also contained a very thick plexus of PSA-NCAM-positive nerve fibres and sparse cell bodies (Figure 10G) and a discrete number of BDNF-positive neurons (Figure 10H). In the upper medulla and pons, a moderate immunostaining for both markers occurred in the main vestibular nuclei, where positive perikarya and nerve fibre networks could be observed at all ages examined (Figure 10E, F).

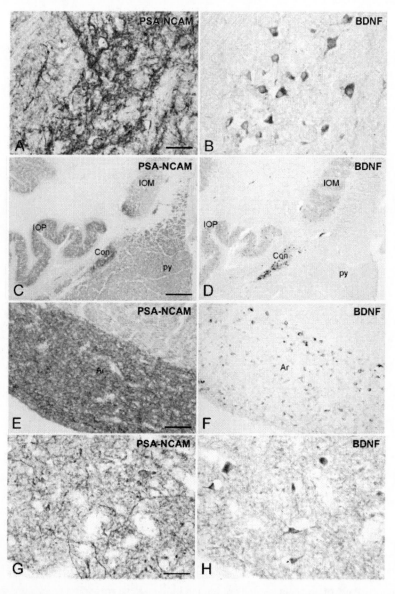

Figure 10. Human pre-term newborn medulla oblongata and pons (case 6). Pairs of adjacent sections immunostained for PSA-NCAM (A, C, E, G) and BDNF (B, D, F, H). A,B: interfascicular nucleus; C,D: left side ventral field showing immunolabelling in the inferior olive principal nucleus (IOP), medial accessory olivary nucleus (IOM) and conterminal nucleus (Con); E,F: arcuate nucleus (Ar); G,H; medial vestibular nucleus. py, pyramidal tract. Scale bars: A, B, G, H = 50 μm; C, D = 500 μm; E, F = 100 μm.

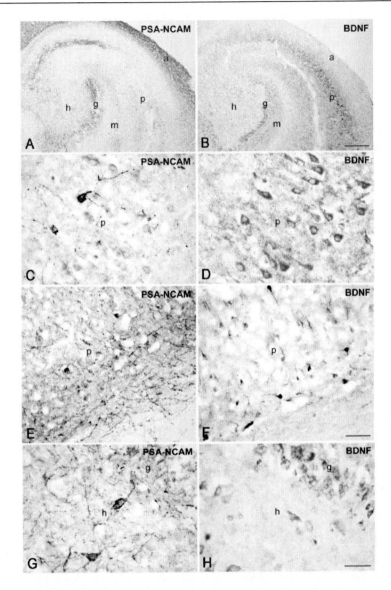

Figure 11. Pairs of adjacent sections of human hippocampal formation from a pre-term newborn (A-D; case 5) and two adult subjects (E,F: case 19; G,H: case 20) immunostained for PSA-NCAM (A, C, E, G) and BDNF (B, D, F, H). A,B: panoramic view of Ammon's horn and fascia dentata; C,D: pyramidal layer, CA2 sector; E,F: pyramidal layer and stratum oriens, CA1 sector; G,H: fascia dentata. g, granular layer; h, hilus; m, molecular layer; o, stratum oriens; p, pyramidal layer. Scale bars: A = B = 500 μm; C = D = E = F = 50 μm; G = H = 20 μm.

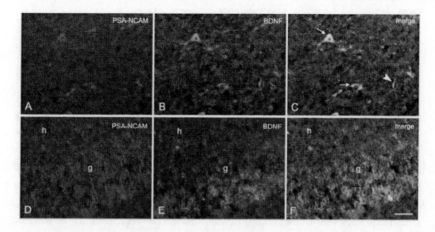

Figure 12. Human hippocampal formation. Immunofluorescence double immunostaining for PSA-NCAM (A, D) and BDNF (B, E) in the fascia dentata of the human pre-term newborn (case 5). C, F: overlay of single immunostainings in A,B and D,E, respectively. Arrows point to double labelled neurons; arrowhead points to a neuron labelled for BDNF alone. Scale bars: A-C, 50 µm; D-F, 20 µm.

In the pons, PSA-NCAM-LI was moderate with the exception of some strongly immunoreactive regions in the territory of the reticulotegmental nucleus. In these regions, a number of BDNF-positive neurons could be observed in the paramedian reticular and pontine reticulotegmental nuclei. The pontine basilar nuclei show numerous BDNF-positive neuronal perikarya. There, PSA-NCAM-LI appeared as a thick punctate PSA-NCAM immunostaining of the neuropil and rare labelled neurons. With few exceptions, for both substances the distribution pattern detected at prenatal age persisted later on, though the immunoreactivity appeared often higher in pre and full-term newborns than in adult specimens.

Hippocampus. Analysis of adjacent sections processed by the avidin-biotin-peroxidase immunohistochemical technique revealed that, at all examined ages, the codistribution of PSA-NCAM- and BDNF-LI occurred throughout (Figure 11). PSA-NCAM-LI appeared mostly as peripheral staining on a number of cell bodies and labelled numerous nerve fibres and terminals, whereas BDNF-LI labelled neuronal perykarya and proximal processes (for a detailed map of BDNF-LI in the human hippocampus at different ages see Quartu et al., 1999).

Analysis of sections double labelled for PSA-NCAM/BDNF, carried out in the pre-term hippocampal formation, revealed the occurrence of PSA-

NCAM-LI and BDNF-LI colocalized in a number of neuronal perikarya, particularly in the hilus of the fascia dentata (Figure 10A-C).

CONCLUSION

The results obtained indicate that in the human nervous system a subpopulation of the TG primary sensory neurons, several regions of the brainstem, and the hippocampal formation express PSA-NCAM throughout life. The distribution pattern of PSA-NCAM-LI is generally conserved from the early prenatal life to adulthood, though age-related changes can be detected in a restricted number of brainstem nuclei and in the hippocampal formation.

Centrally, at the brainstem level, the sialylated protein appears associated with most of the sensory nuclei, in agreement with findings on laboratory animals and the concept that, in these regions, the expression of growth-related proteins may subserve structural reorganization and synaptic plasticity in response to afferent activity (Bonfanti, 2006; Bouzioukh et al., 2001) throughout life (Emery et al., 2003).

As for the spinal trigeminal sensory system, occurrence of the growth-associated protein-43 (GAP-43) has been reported in both the sensory ganglion and the central nuclei (Del Fiacco et al., 1994). The localization of PSA-NCAM to the caudal part of the trigeminal spinal sensory nucleus and its changes with age are consistent with data on the dorsal horn of the rat spinal cord, showing that PSA-NCAM is more widely expressed during embryonic and early postnatal than in adult life, when it is confined to the superficial laminae (Bonfanti et al., 1992; Seki et al., 1993b). Such a discrete central localization of the molecule together with the morphometric characteristics of the immunoreactive trigeminal primary sensory neurons point to an involvement of PSA-NCAM in the functional roles of neurotransmission and processing of protopathic sensory stimuli.

It is interesting that a PSA-dependent reversible loss of C terminals occurs in the spinal lamina II in a model of chronic neuropathic pain (El Maarouf et al., 2005). In this context, it has been proposed that, under injury or stress conditions, the presence of PSA allows for a local and reversible break in the afferent pathway in response to excessive stimulation, and thereby could serve to protect central circuitry from chronic sensory overload (El Maarouf et al., 2005).

PSA-NCAM has been shown in the chicken acoustic ganglion cells (Kajikawa et al., 1997), where a role for the molecule in neuronal plasticity and in the processing of auditory information has been suggested. Afferents to the mouse ventral cochlear nucleus express high levels of PSA (El Maarouf et al., 2005) and, similarly to the structural plasticity of nociceptive C terminals in chronic neuropathic pain (El Maarouf et al., 2005), it has been reported that noxious acoustic insults are associated with a reversible atrophy of nerve terminals in the ventral cochlear nucleus (Bilak et al., 1997; Kim et al., 1997; Morest et al., 1997).

Our observations also indicate that at all ages examined the dorsal vagal complex, namely the nucleus of the solitary tract, the dorsal motor nucleus of the vagus nerve, and the area postrema, contains PSA-NCAM-labelled neurons, nerve fibres and terminals. A convergent set of experimental data shows that in these areas, though visceral sensorimotor circuits are morphologically established in newborn rats (Rinaman et al., 1993; Cheng et al., 2004), intense dynamic changes of neuronal properties still occur after birth (Bouzioukh et al., 2001; Takemura et al., 1996; Vincent et al., 1996; 1997; 1999; Rao et al., 1997; Moyse et al., 2006).

In the rat solitary tract nucleus, the overall PSA-NCAM expression decreases during the first two postnatal weeks and persists only at synapses in the adult (Bouzioukh et al., 2001). Furthermore, PSA-NCAM expression has been shown to be dynamically controlled by the electrical stimulation of the vagal afferents (Bouzioukh et al., 2001) and, conversely, a repetitive stimulation of afferent fibres leads to phasic and long-term plasticity in adult animals (Zhou et al., 1997). It has been shown that the rat raphe serotonin neurons do not express PSA-NCAM (Brezun et al., 1999). Thus, it may be considered that the staining on the raphe neuronal perikarya observed in our specimens either belongs to those neurons, marking a difference with the rat species, or reflects the occurrence of positive elements impinging on the raphe neuronal somata.

PSA-NCAM occurs in most of the precerebellar nuclei, which act as a gate for the input to the cerebellum. Its expression appears particularly robust in nuclei which play a critical role in eye movement control, such as the perihypoglossal nuclei and the paramedian reticular nucleus (Hopp et al., 2004; Tilikete et al., 2008; Quartu et al., 2010).

PSA-NCAM-related neuroplasticity may also involve glial cells. Several lines of evidence indicate that PSA-NCAM plays a permissive role for the structural remodelling of neuronal and glial cells, particularly in the neuroendocrine system, where PSA-NCAM appears to control the retraction of the glial processes in the hypothalamo-neurohypophysial system (Bonfanti, 2006; Parkash et al., 2007). Moreover, changes in PSA-NCAM in the avian ciliary ganglion after axonal injury also involve perineuronal satellite cells (De Stefano et al., 2001). In agreement with the steric hindrance caused by the molecule (Rutishauser, 2008; Johnson et al., 2005), the occurrence of PSA-NCAM in the TG may indicate sites of detachment between the neuronal surface and its glial ensheatment. Dynamic changes, such as remodelling of the perikaryal surface, that may be operated via other growth-related proteins such as GAP-43 (Nacimiento et al., 1993), may be facilitated by this effect.

As for the finding of PSA-NCAM-positive ependymal cells in the central canal lining, it is possible that we are observing a subpopulation of glial cells which, during gestation and up to early infancy, remain undifferentiated as potential neural progenitor cells, as recently suggested in the human brain (Sakakibara et al., 2007).

PSA-NCAM is highly expressed in the human hippocampus under normal conditions supporting the concept that this area of the human brain, known for its role in memory formation, undergoes continuous remodelling throughout life. Previous studies have focussed on the presence and persistence of PSA-NCAM from infancy (5 months) and adolescence (8 years) (Ni Dhuill et al., 1999) to adult life (Ní Dhúill et al., 1999; Mikkonen et al., 1999; Arellano et al., 2003). The present results are in agreement with the tissue distribution of PSA-NCAM in the hippocampus and show further that PSA-NCAM can be detected in this region from prenatal life, as early as 21 w.g., to the full-term age. One of the most interesting observations is the presence of PSA-NCAM-LI in the granule cell layer and its persistence in cells at the granular layer/hilar border.

In the rodent, these cells have been suggested to represent newborn granule cell precursors (Seki et al., 1993a). However, in human hippocampus infragranular cells have been shown to be quite heterogeneous with respect to their morphology, dendritic projections, and electrophysiological response (Amaral, 1978; Mott et al., 1997), suggesting that in this region the persistence of PSA-NCAM-LI throughout lifespan may reflect their involvement in functions other than neurogenesis. The neurochemical characterization and connectivity of the PSA-NCAM-positive neurons is an important issue and deserves further investigation. The concurrent presence of PSA-NCAM and BDNF in several brainstem nuclei and hippocampal formation suggests that PSA-NCAM, besides signalling *per se* dynamic events related to neuroplasticity, may also act as interface between BDNF and its receptors.

In fact, it has been proposed that PSA-NCAM can promote the "cis" clustering of trkB and help the ligand–receptor interaction by increasing the local concentration of BDNF in the vicinity of trkB, thus facilitating its ligand-mediated activation (Kiss et al., 2001; Bonfanti, 2006). This possibility appears particularly plausible in hippocampal neurons where colocalization of PSA-NCAM/BDNF is detectable (present results). Moreover, PSA-NCAM has been reported to be able to inhibit the expression of p75 (Gascon et al., 2007), thus modulating the effects mediated by the low affinity neurotrophin receptor (Bredesen et al., 2005; Waterhouse et al., 2009). Interestingly, neuronal populations of Ammon's horn and fascia dentata express several neurotrophic factors and relevant tyrosine-kinase receptors (Serra et al., 2002a; 2002b; 2005; Quartu et al., 1999; 2005; Webster et al., 2006), among which is glial cell line-derived neurotrophic factor (GDNF) which has been shown to stimulate hippocampal axonal growth via binding to NCAM and activation of Fyn (Paratcha et al., 2003; 2008; Sjöstrand et al., 2007).

ACKNOWLEDGMENTS

MQ and MDF acknowledge research funding by the University of Cagliari and the Fondazione Banco di Sardegna.

REFERENCES

Angata, K. and Fukuda, M. Polysialyltransferases: major players in polysialic acid synthesis on the neural cell adhesion molecule. *Biochimie* 2003, 85, 195-206.

Arellano, J. I., DeFelipe, J., Muñoz, A. PSA-NCAM immunoreactivity in chandelier cell axon terminals of the human temporal cortex. *Cereb. Cortex* 2002, 12, 617-624.

Barbeau, D., Liang, J. J., Robitalille, Y., Quirion, R., Srivastava, L. K. Decreased expression of the embryonic form of the neural cell adhesion molecule in schizophrenic brains. *Proc. Natl. Acad. Sci. US* 1995, 92, 2785-2789.

Becker, C. G., Artola, A., Gerardy-Schahn, R., Becker, T., Welzl, H., Schachner, M. The polysialic acid modification of the neural cell adhesion molecule is involved in spatial learning and hippocampal long-term potentiation. *J. Neurosci. Res.* 1996, 45, 143-152.

Bilak, M., Kim, J., Potashner, S. J., Bohne, B. A., Morest, D. K. New growth of axons in the cochlear nucleus of adult chinchillas after acoustic trauma. *Exp. Neurol.* 1997, 147, 256-268.

Bonfanti, L. PSA-NCAM in mammalian structural plasticity and neurogenesis. *Prog. Neurobiol.* 2006, 80, 129-164.

Bonfanti, L., Merighi, A., Theodosis, D. T. Dorsal rhizotomy induces transient expression of the highly sialylated isoform of the neural cell adhesion molecule in neurons and astrocytes of the adult rat spinal cord. *Neuroscience* 1996, 74, 619-623.

Bonfanti, L., Olive, S., Poulain, D. A., Theodosis, D. T. Mapping of the distribution of polysialylated neural cell adhesion molecule throughout the central nervous system of the adult rat: an immunohistochemical study. *Neuroscience* 1992, 49, 418-436.

Bouzioukh, F., Tell, F., Rougon, G., Jean, A. Dual effects of NMDA receptor activation on polysialylated neural cell adhesion molecule expression during brainstem postnatal development. *Eur. J. Neurosci.* 2001, 14, 1194-1202.

Bredesen, D. E., Mehlen, P., Rabizadeh, S. Receptors that mediate cellular dependence. *Cell Death Differ.* 2005, 12, 1031–1043.

Brezun, J. M. and Daszuta, A. Serotonin depletion in the adult rat produces differential changes in highly polysialylated form of neural cell adhesion molecule and tenascin-C immunoreactivity. *J. Neurosci. Res.* 1999, 55, 54-70.

Charles, P., Reynolds, R., Seilhean, D., Rougon, G., Aigrot, M. S., Niezgoda, A., Zalc, B., Lubetzki, C. Re-expression of PSA-NCAM by demyelinated axons: an inhibitor of remyelination in multiple sclerosis? *Brain* 2002, 125, 1972-1979.

Cheng, G., Zhou, X., Qu, J., Ashwell, K. W., Paxinos, G. Central vagal sensory and motor connections: human embryonic and fetal development. *Auton. Neurosci.* 2004, 114, 83-96.

De Stefano, M. E., Leone, L., Paggi, P. Polysialylated neural cell adhesion molecule is involved in the neuroplasticity induced by axonal injury in the avian ciliary ganglion. *Neuroscience* 2001, 103, 1093-1104.

Del Fiacco, M., Quartu, M., Priestley, J. V., Setzu, M. D., Lai, M. L. GAP-43 persists in adulthood and coexists with SP and CGRP in human trigeminal sensory neurones. *Neuroreport* 1994, 5, 2349-2352.

Dubois, C., Figarella-Branger, D., Pastoret, C., Rampini, C., Karpati, G., Rougon, G. Expression of NCAM and its polysialylated isoforms during mdx mouse muscle regeneration and in vitro myogenesis. *Neuromuscul. Disord.* 1994, 4, 171-182.

Duveau, V., Arthaud, S., Rougier, A., Le Gal La Salle, G. Polysialylation of NCAM is upregulated by hyperthermia and participates in heat shock preconditioning-induced neuroprotection. *Neurobiol. Disease* 2007, 26, 385-395.

El Maarouf, A. and Rutishauser, U. Removal of polysialic acid induces aberrant pathways, synaptic vesicle distribution, and terminal arborization of retinotectal axons. *J. Comp. Neurol.* 2003, 460, 203-211.

El Maarouf, A. and Rutishauser, U. Use of PSA-NCAM in repair of the Central Nervous System. *Neurochem. Res.* 2008.

El Maarouf, A., Kolesnikov, Y., Pasternak, G., Rutishauser, U. Polysialic acid-induced plasticity reduces neuropathic insult to the central nervous system. *Proc. Natl. Acad. Sci. US* 2005, 102, 11516-11520.

El Maarouf, A., Petridis, A. K., Rutishauser, U. Use of polysialic acid in repair of the central nervous system. *Proc. Natl. Acad. Sci. US* 2006, 103, 16989-16994.

Emery, D. L., Royo, N. C., Fischer, I., Saatman, K. E., McIntosh, T. K. Plasticity following injury to the adult nervous system: is recapitulation of a developmental state worth promoting? *J. Neurotrauma* 2003, 20, 1271-1292.

Fox, G. B., Fichera, G., Barry, T., O'Connell, A. W., Gallagher, H. C., Murphy, K. J., Regan, C. M. Consolidation of passive avoidance learning is associated with transient increases of polysialylated neurons in layer II of the rat medial temporal cortex. *J. Neurobiol.* 2000, 45, 145-141.

Franz, C. K., Rutishauser, U., Rafuse, V. F. Polysialylated neural cell adhesion molecule is necessary for selective targeting of regenerating motor neurons. *J. Neurosci.* 2005, 25, 2081-2091.

Gascon, E., Vutskits, L., Jenny, B., Durbec, P., Kiss, J. Z. PSA-NCAM in postnatally generated immature neurons of the olfactory bulb: a crucial role in regulating p75 expression and cell survival. *Development* 2007, 134, 1181-1190.

Hopp, J. J. and Fuchs, A. F. The characteristics and neuronal substrate of saccadic eye movement plasticity. *Prog. Neurobiol.* 2004, 72, 27-53.

Iwai, M., Hayashi, T., Zhang, W. R., Sato, K., Manabe, Y., Abe, K. Induction of highly polysialylated neuronal cell adhesion molecule (PSA-NCAM) in postischemic gerbil hippocampus mainly dissociated with neural stem cell proliferation. *Brain Res.* 2001, 902, 288-293.

Jakovcevski, I., Mo, Z., Zecevic, N. Down-regulation of the axonal polysialic acid-neural cell adhesion molecule expression coincides with the onset of myelination in the human fetal forebrain. *Neuroscience* 2007, 149, 328-337.

Johnson, C. P., Fujimoto, I., Rutishauser, U., Leckband, D. E. Direct evidence that neural cell adhesion molecule (NCAM) polysialylation increases intermembrane repulsion and abrogates adhesion. *J. Biol. Chem.* 2005, 280, 137-145. Erratum in: *J. Biol. Chem.* 2005, 280, 23424.

Kajikawa, H., Umemoto, M., Mishiro, Y., Sakagami, M., Kubo, T., Yoneda, Y. Expression of highly polysialylated NCAM (NCAM-H) in developing and adult chicken auditory organ. *Hearing Res.* 1997, 203, 123-130.

Kim, J., Morest, D. K., Bohne, B. A. Degeneration of axons in the brainstem of the chinchilla after auditory overstimulation. *Hear. Res.* 1997, 103, 169-191.

Kiss, J. Z. and Rougon, G. Cell biology of polysialic acid. *Curr. Opin. Neurobiol.* 1997, 7, 640-646.

Kiss, J. Z., Troncoso, E., Djebbara, Z., Vutskits, L., Muller, D. The role of neural cell adhesion molecules in plasticity and repair. *Brain Res. Rev.* 2001, 36, 175–184.

Luzzati, F., Bonfanti, L., Fasolo, A., Peretto, P. DCX and PSA-NCAM expression identifies a population of neurons preferentially distributed in associative areas of different pallial derivatives and vertebrate species. *Cereb. Cortex.* 2009, 19, 1028-1041.

Mathern, G. W., Leiphart, J. L., De Vera, A., Adelson, P. D., Seki, T., Neder, L., Leite, J. P. Seizures decrease postnatal neurogenesis and granule cell development in the human fascia dentata. *Epilepsia* 2002, 43 (Suppl. 5), 68-73.

Mikkonen, M., Soininen, H., Kälviänen, R., Tapiola, T., Ylinen, A., Vapalahti, M., Paljärvi, L., Pitkänen, A. Remodeling of neuronal circuitries in human temporal lobe epilepsy: increased expression of highly polysialylated neural cell adhesion molecule in the hippocampus and the entorhinal cortex. *Ann. Neurol.* 1998, 44, 923-934.

Mikkonen, M., Soininen, H., Tapiola, T., Alafuzoff, I., Miettinen, R. Hippocampal plasticity in Alzheimer's disease: changes in highly polysialylated NCAM immunoreactivity in the hippocampal formation. *Eur. J. Neurosci.* 1999, 11, 1754-1764.

Morest, D. K., Kim, J., Bohne, B. A. Neuronal and transneuronal degeneration of auditory axons in the brainstem after cochlear lesions in the chinchilla: cochleotopic and non-cochleotopic patterns. *Hear. Res.* 1997, 103, 151-168.

Moyse, E., Baner, S., Charrier, C., Coronas, V., Krantic, S., Jean, A. Neurogenesis and neural stem cells in the dorsal vagal complex of adult rat brain: new vistas about autonomic regulations-a review. *Autonom. Neurosci.* 2006, 126-127, 50-58.

Muller, D., Djebbara-Hannas, Z., Jourdain, P., Vutskits, L., Durbec, P., Rougon, G., Kiss, J. Z. Brain-derived neurotrophic factor restores long term potentiation in polysialic acid-neural cell adhesion molecule-deficient hippocampus. *Proc. Natl. Acad. Sci. US.* 2000, 97, 4315-4320.

Muller, D., Wang, C., Skibo, G. PSA-NCAM is required for activity-induced synaptic plasticity. *Neuron* 1996, 17, 413-422.

Nacher, J., Pham, K., Gil-Fernandez, V., McEwen, B. S. Chronic restraint stress and chronic corticosterone treatment modulate differentially the expression of molecules related to structural plasticity in the adult rat piriform cortex. *Neuroscience* 2004, 126, 503-509.

Nacimiento, W., Töpper, R., Fischer, A., Oestreicher, A. B., Nacimiento, A. C., Gispen, W. H., Noth, J., Kreutzberg, G. W. Immunocytochemistry of B-50 (GAP-43) in the spinal cord and in dorsal root ganglia of the adult cat. *J. Neurocytol.* 1993, 22, 413-424.

Nguyen, L., Rigo, J. M., Malgrange, B., Moonen, G., Belachew, S. Untangling the functional potential of PSA-NCAM-expressing cells in CNS development and brain repair strategies. *Curr. Med. Chem.* 2003, 10, 2185-2196.

Ní Dhúill, C. M., Fox, G. B., Pittock, S. J., O'Connell, A. W., Murphy, K. J., Regan, C. M. Polysialylated neural cell adhesion molecule expression in the dentate gyrus of the human hippocampal formation from infancy to old age. *J. Neurosci. Res.* 1999, 55, 99-106.

Paratcha, G. and Ledda, F. GDNF and GFRalpha: a versatile molecular complex for developing neurons. *Trends Neurosci.* 2008, 31, 384-391.

Paratcha, G., Ledda, F., Ibanez, C. F. The neural cell adhesion melecula NCAM is an alternative signaling receptor for GDNF family ligands. *Cell* 2003, 113, 814-825.

Parkash, J. and Kaur, G. Potential of PSA-NCAM in neuron-glial plasticity in the adult hypothalamus: role of noradrenergic and GABAergic neurotransmitters. *Brain Res. Bull.* 2007, 74, 317-328.

Pham, K., Nacher, J., Hof, P. R., McEwen, B. S. Repeated restraint stress suppresses neurogenesis and induces biphasic PSA-NCAM expression in the adult rat dentate gyrus. *Eur. J. Neurosci.* 2003, 17, 879-886.

Quartu, M., Lai, M. L., Del Fiacco, M. Neurotrophin-like immunoreactivity in the human hippocampal formation. *Brain Res. Bull.* 1999, 48, 375-382.

Quartu, M., Serra, M. P., Boi, M., Ibba, V., Melis, T., Del Fiacco, M. Polysialylated-neural cell adhesion molecule (PSA-NCAM) in the human trigeminal ganglion and brainstem at prenatal and adult ages. *BMC Neurosci.* 2008, 9, 108.

Quartu, M., Serra, M. P., Boi, M., Melis, T., Ambu, R., Del Fiacco, M. Brain-derived neurotrophic factor (BDNF) and polysialylated-neural cell adhesion molecule (PSA-NCAM): codistribution in the human brainstem precerebellar nuclei from prenatal to adult age. *Brain Res.* 2010, 1363, 49-62.

Quartu, M., Serra, M. P., Manca, A., Mascia, F., Follesa, P., Del Fiacco, M. Neurturin, persephin, and artemin in the human pre- and full-term newborn and adult hippocampus and fascia dentata. *Brain Res.* 2005, 1041, 157-166.

Rao, H., Pio, J., Kessler, J. P. Postnatal ontogeny of glutamate receptors in the rat nucleus tractus solitarii and ventrolateral medulla. *J. Auton. Nerv. Syst.* 1999, 65, 25-32.

Rinaman, L. and Levitt, P. Establishment of vagal sensorimotor circuits during fetal development in rats. *J. Neurobiol.* 1993, 24, 641-659.

Roche, P.-H., Figarella-Branger, D., Daniel, L., Bianco, N., Pellet, W., Pellissier, J.-F. Expression of cell adhesion molecules in normal nerves, chronic axonal neuropathies and Schwann cell tumors. *J. Neurol. Sci.* 1997, 151, 127-133.

Ronn, L. C., Berezin, V., Bock, E. The neural cell adhesion molecule in synaptic plasticity and ageing. *Int. J. Dev. Neurosci.* 2000, 18, 193-199.

Rutishauser, U. and Landmesser, L. Polysialic acid in the vertebrate nervous system: a promoter of plasticity in cell-cell interactions. *Trends Neurosci.* 1996, 19, 422-427.

Rutishauser, U. Polysialic acid in the plasticity of the developing and adult vertebrate nervous system. *Nature* 2008, 9, 26-35.

Sakakibara, A., Aoki, E., Hashizume, Y., Mori, N., Nakayama, A. Distribution of nestin and other stem cell-related molecules in developing and diseased human spinal cord. *Pathol. Int.* 2007, 57, 358-568.

Sandi, C., Merino, J. J., Cordero, M. L., Kruyt, N. D., Murphy, K. J., Regan, C. M. Modulation of hippocampal NCAM polysialylation and spatial memory consolidation by fear conditioning. *Biol. Psychiatry* 2003, 54, 599-607.

Seki, Y. and Arai, T. Distribution and possible roles of highly polysialylated neural cell adhesion molecule (NCAM-H) in the developing and adult central nervous system. *Neurosci. Res.* 1993a, 17, 265-290.

Seki, Y. and Arai, T.: Highly polysialylated NCAM expression in the developing and adult rat spinal cord. *Dev. Brain Res.* 1993b, 73:141-145.

Serra, M. P., Quartu, M., Ambu, R., Follesa, P., Del Fiacco, M. Immunohistochemical localization of GDNF in the human hippocampal formation from prenatal life to adulthood. *Brain Res.* 2002a, 928, 138-146.

Serra, M. P., Quartu, M., Lai, M. L., Follesa, P., Del Fiacco, M. Expression of glial cell line-derived neurotrophic factor mRNA in the human newborn and adult hippocampal formation. *Brain Res.* 2002b, 928, 160-164.

Serra, M. P., Quartu, M., Mascia, F., Manca, A., Boi, M., Pisu, M. G., Lai, M. L., Del Fiacco, M. Ret, GFRalpha-1, GFRalpha-2 and GFRalpha-3 receptors in the human hippocampus and fascia dentata. *Int. J. Dev. Neurosci.* 2005, 23, 425-438.

Singh, J. and Kaur, G. Neuroprotection mediated by subtoxic dose of NMDA and SH-SY5Y neuroblastoma cultures: activity-dependent regulation of PSA-NCAM expression. *Mol. Brain Res.* 2005, 137, 223-234.

Sjöstrand, D., Carlsson, J., Paratcha, G., Persson, B., Ibáñez, C. F. Disruption of the GDNF binding site in NCAM dissociates ligand binding and homophilic cell adhesion. *J. Biol. Chem.* 2007, 282, 12734-12740.

Takemura, M., Wakisaka, S., Iwase, K., Yabuta, N. H., Nakagawa, S., Chen, K., Bae, Y. C., Yoshida, A., Shigenaga, Y. NADPH-diaphorase in the developing rat: lower brainstem and cervical spinal cord, with special reference to the trigemino-solitary complex. *J. Comp. Neurol.* 1996, 365, 511-525.

Theodosis, D. T., Bonhomme, R., Vitiello, S., Rougon, G., Poulain, D. A. Cell surface expression of polysialic acid on NCAM is a prerequisite for activity-dependent morphological neuronal and glial plasticity. *J. Neurosci.* 1999, 19, 10228-10236.

Tilikete, C. and Pélisson, D. Ocular motor syndromes of the brainstem and cerebellum. *Curr. Opin. Neurol.* 2008, 21, 22-28.

Ulfig, N. and Chan, W. Y., Expression patterns of PSA-NCAM in the human ganglionic eminence and its vicinity: role of PSA-NCAM in neuronal migration and axonal growth? *Cells Tissues Organs* 2004, 177, 229-236.

Varea, E., Castillo-Gómez, E., Gómez-Climent, M. A., Blasco-Ibáñez, J. M., Crespo, C., Martínez-Guijarro, F. J., Nàcher, J. PSA-NCAM expression in the human prefrontal cortex. *J. Chem. Neuroanat.* 2007, 33, 202-209.

Varea, E., Guirado, R., Gilabert-Juan, J., Martí, U., Castillo-Gomez, E., Blasco-Ibáñez, J. M., Crespo, C., Nacher, J. Expression of PSA-NCAM and synaptic proteins in the amygdala of psychiatric disorder patients. *J. Psychiatr. Res.* 2012, 46, 189-197.

Vincent, A, Jean, A, Tell, F. Developmental study of N-methyl-D-aspartate-induced firing activity and whole-cell currents in nucleus tractus solitarii neurons. *Eur. J. Neurosci.* 1996, 8, 2748-2752.

Vincent, A. and Tell, F. Postnatal changes in electrophysiological properties of rat nucleus tractus solitarii neurons. *Eur. J. Neurosci.* 1997, 9, 1612-1624.

Vincent, A. and Tell, F. Postnatal development of rat nucleus tractus solitarius neurons: morphological and electrophysiological evidence. *Neuroscience* 1999, 93, 293-305.

Vutskits, L., Djebbara-Hannas, Z., Zhang, H., Paccaud, J. P., Durbec, P., Rougon, G., Muller, D., Kiss, J. Z. PSA-NCAM modulates BDNF-dependent survival and differentiation of cortical neurons. *Eur. J. Neurosci.* 2001, 13, 1391-1402.

Vutskits, L., Gascon, E., Kiss, J. Z. Removal of PSA from NCAM affects the survival of magnocellular vasopressin- and oxytocin-producing neurons in organotypic cultures of the paraventricular nucleus. *Eur. J. Neurosci.* 2003, 17, 2119-2126.

Waterhouse, E. G. and Xu, B. New insights into the role of brain-derived neurotrophic factor in synaptic plasticity. *Mol. Cell. Neurosci.* 2009, 42, 81–89.

Weber, M., Modemann, S., Schipper, P., Trauer, H., Franke, H., Illes, P., Geiger, K. D., Hengstler, J. G., Kleemann, W. J. Increased polysialic acid neural cell adhesion molecule expression in human hippocampus of heroin addicts. *Neuroscience* 2006, 138, 1215-1223.

Webster, M. J., Herman, M. M., Kleinman, J. E., ShannonWeickert, C. S. BDNF and trkB mRNA expression in the hippocampus and temporal cortex during the human lifespan. *Gene Expr. Patterns* 2006, 6, 941–951.

Zhou, Z., Champagnat, J., Poon, C.-S. Phasic and long-term depression in brainstem nucleus tractus solitarius neurons: differing roles of AMPA receptor desensitization. *J. Neurosci.* 1997, 17, 5349-5356.

Reviewed by Prof. John Priestley,

Centre for Neuroscience and Trauma, Barts and The London School of Medicine and Dentistry, Queen Mary University of London.

In: Recent Advances in Adhesions Research   ISBN: 978-1-62417-447-6
Editors: A. McFarland and M. Akins   © 2013 Nova Science Publishers, Inc.

Chapter 3

AN OVERVIEW IN SURGICAL ADHESIVES

*P. Ferreira, M. H. Gil and P. Alves**

University of Coimbra, Department of
Chemical Engineering, Portugal

ABSTRACT

A wound may be defined as an injury to any of the body's tissues, especially one caused by physical means and with interruption of continuity.

Primary wound healing of a plan-to-plan oriented scar formation is usually accomplished by hand sewing or stapling the corresponding layers of each side of the incision. Both these methods have been associated to wound infection and granule formation due to their degradation in the organism. They also present other disadvantages, such as the need to be removed (in most cases) and the pain associated with their use.

As a result of these shortcomings, surgeons have thought of an alternative way: the use of medical tissue adhesives. These adhesives consist on an attractive option to suturing or stapling since they can accomplish other tasks, such as haemostasis and the ability of sealing air leakages and also because they do not represent any risk of needlestick injury to medical staff. Also, the use of an adhesive would reduce the surgeries procedure time since its application presents itself as an easier and faster method to establish tissue adhesion.

---

* Corresponding author: P. Alves. E-mail: palves@eq.uc.pt.

Despite their advantages, surgical adhesives must obey some clinical requirements. They must hold the two sides of the tissue together until it is no longer necessary, and then they should be degraded to biocompatible products.

The most used surgical glues nowadays are the fibrin based adhesives and cyanoacrylates. Fibrin based adhesives present several problems, e.g. immunogenicity and risk of blood transmission diseases such as HIV and BSE. On the other hand, cyanoacrylates have been reported to degrade in aqueous media producing formaldehyde, which causes inflammation and has carcinogenic potential. Other options are now coming into light, and among the synthetic materials, urethane-based adhesives have been considered to be the most promising. These materials may be prepared under the form of pre-polymers (containing free isocyanate groups) and therefore being able to react with amino groups present in the biological molecules establishing adhesion. Another current area of research is the synthesis of UV-curable adhesives. These offer major advantages compared to pre-polymers systems, such as fast-curing rate, control of polymerization heat evolution and are ideal for application to weakened and diseased tissue.

Throughout this chapter, examples of currently applied bioadhesives in surgery, as well as their advantages and disadvantages will be described. A special emphasis will be given to the development of polyurethane based adhesives both in the pre-polymer and UV-curable forms.

Keywords: Surgical adhesives, fibrin, cyanoacrylates, urethanes

1. INTRODUCTION

The need for materials, which allow the healing of the human body, is as old as the medicine itself. The eldest known reference related with surgical intervention on traumatic wounds is the Edwin Smith Papyrus, an Ancient Egyptian medical text, dating from the XVII century B.C. (Atta, 1999). The author recommended the use of suture strands for open wound closure.

In fact, even nowadays, stitching and stapling are the most common and popular procedures in wound closure. Both of them have been associated to wound infection and granule formation due to their degradation in the organism.

They also present other disadvantages, such as the need to be removed, in most cases, and the pain associated with their application. As a result of these shortcomings, surgeons have thought as an alternative way, the use of medical tissue adhesives.

Nowadays, topical skin adhesives are beginning to be largely used by health professionals to replace sutures and staples since they present several vantages. Among them it is possible to highlight the fact that they are less traumatic, do not require anaesthesia and may accomplish other tasks, such as haemostasis and the ability of sealing air leakages.

Also, unlike staples or stitches (if not degradable), they do not need to be further removal and usually allow obtaining excellent cosmetic results. Finally, tissue adhesives also present the potential to work as delivery systems and can be engineered for slow, localized release of medications, such as pain treatment drugs, antibiotics or chemotherapy treatment.

However, surgical adhesives must obey some clinical requirements. They must hold the two sides of the tissue together while necessary, and then they should be degraded to biocompatible products (Lipatova, 1986).

Among the materials which have already been testedwhose usehas already been testedinclinical trials are the cyanoacrylates, fibrin,gelatin-crosslinkedadhesives(gelatin/resorcinol/formaldehyde), polyethylene glycolhydrogels, proteins such as collagen, silk, elastin and other derived mucins and also somepolyurethanes. Some of these materialsare describedin subsequent sections of this chapter.

2. ADHESIVES IN SURGERY

A biological adhesive must combine three major characteristics: biocompatibility, performance and effectiveness. Besides, it should also present a fast curing rate when in contact with the living tissues.

Surgical adhesives need to follow some clinical requirements, such as: hold the two sides of the tissue together, until needed, and should degrade to biocompatible products (Lipatova, 1986).

Several natural substances may be used as bioadhesives, being proteins and carbohydrates the most used ones. For many years, proteins such as gelatin and carbohydrates such as starch have been used as general-purpose glues, but due to their performance limitations they have been replaced by synthetic alternatives.

Nowadays, the most used surgical glues are fibrin based adhesives (Albala, 2003) and cyanoacrylates (Eaglstein and Sullivan, 2005). Fibrin based adhesives have several problems, such as immunogenicity and risk of blood transmission diseases such as HIV and BSE. On the other hand, cyanoacrylates have been reported to degrade in aqueous media to produce formaldehyde, which causes inflammation and have carcinogenicity potential.

2.1. Synthetic Adhesives

Although both natural and synthetic polymers have already been used in the preparation of tissue adhesives, there are some advantages in using synthetic macromolecules.

In general terms, when polymers are man-made, it becomes possible to control some aspects of polymer structure that allow producing tailor-made materials suitable to the desired biological application. Also, three-dimensional structure as well as chemical composition can be controlled in order to adjust materials properties and orientation of specific functional groups that can interact with biological tissues.

However, molecular weight of non-biodegradable synthetic polymers must be well known. Since these polymers must be eliminated by the kidneys, they should present a uniform molecular weight distribution that fits under the threshold of renal excretion (Kabanov and Okano, 2001).

For many years, polymers with the ability to adhere to both hard and soft tissue have been used in surgery and dentistry. Currently, the majority of synthetic bioadhesive polymers are polyacrylic acid derivatives (carbopol, polycarbophil, polyacrylic acid, (PAAc), polyacrylate, poly (methylvinylether-co-methacrylate), poly (methacrylate), poly (acrylcyanoacrylate), poly (isohexylcyanoacrylate), and poly (isobutylcyanocrylate)) and cellulose derivatives (carboxymethyl cellulose, sodium carboxymethyl cellulose, methyl cellulose, and methylhydroxyethyl cellulose) (Patel, 2010).

Synthetic based-materials such as cyanoacrylates, usually act by closing the wound by overlapping the incision ends.

On the other hand, biological based products, like collagen or fibrin glues have intrinsic haemostatic properties that help in the coagulation process (Busuttil, 2003). Table I shows the main applications of surgical adhesives in medicine (PPTI, 2000).

Several materials have been tested in the medical field, among them cyanoacrylates, polyethylene glycol hydrogels, fibrin, crosslinked gelatin (gelatin/resorcinol/formaldehyde), collagen, silk, elastin and other mucin-derived proteins. Some of these biomaterials will be further described through the next sections.

Table1. Main applications of surgical adhesives in medicine

SURGICAL FIELD	Control of haemostasis	Control of air or fluids leakage
Cardiac surgery	X	
General surgery		X
Cirurgia geral (fígado)	X	
Gynecological surgery	X	
Neurosurgery	X	X
Cirurgia ortopédica	X	
Plastic surgery	X	
Thoracic surgery (lung)		X
Urological surgery	X	X

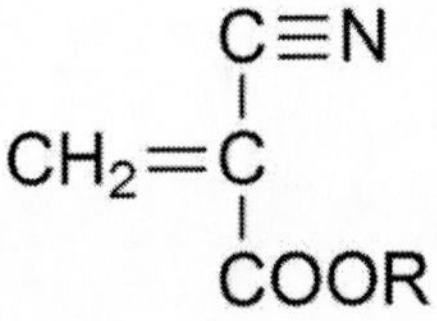

$$CH_2 = \underset{\underset{COOR}{|}}{\overset{\overset{C \equiv N}{|}}{C}}$$

Figure 1. Chemical structure of cyanoacrylate monomer (where R=Alkyl group).

2.1.1. Cyanoacrylate Adhesives

Due to their high adhesion capacity, cyanoacrylates were the first material used as a surgical adhesive, introduced by Ardis (1949). The fast polymerization reaction of these materials and their strong adhesion properties to surfaces have made them one the most used and studied synthetic surgical adhesive in the medical field (Kopecek e Ulbrich, 1983). Cyanoacrylates are synthetic glues that polymerize quickly when in contact with water or blood (Seewald, 2002). Cyanoacrylate monomers can be chemically represented by the structure presented in Figure 1.

When polymerized, the chemical structure of the obtained compound can be represented as shown on Figure 2.

Cyanoacrylates are polymerized in the presence of a weak base, like water, establishing strong bonds with lower elasticity and releasing heat (exothermic reaction). According to some authors (Woodward, 1965), this heat release is relatedtosize of the alkyl group: the smaller the group, the higher the heat release. Besides this heat release, further studies made with methyl 2-cyanoacrylate proved that this adhesive was associated with a high toxicity level.

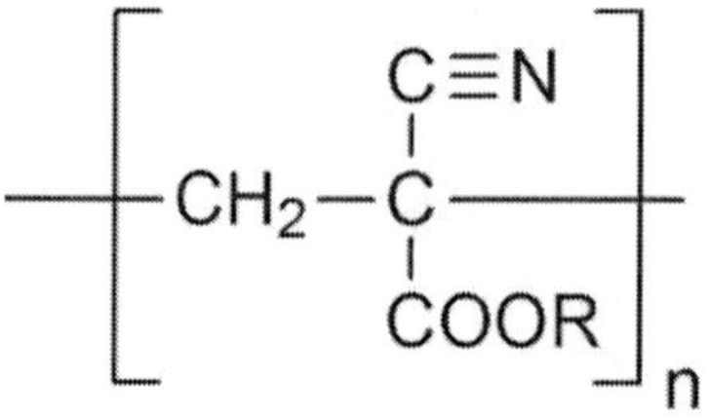

Figure 2. Representation of the structural unit of cyanoacrylates.

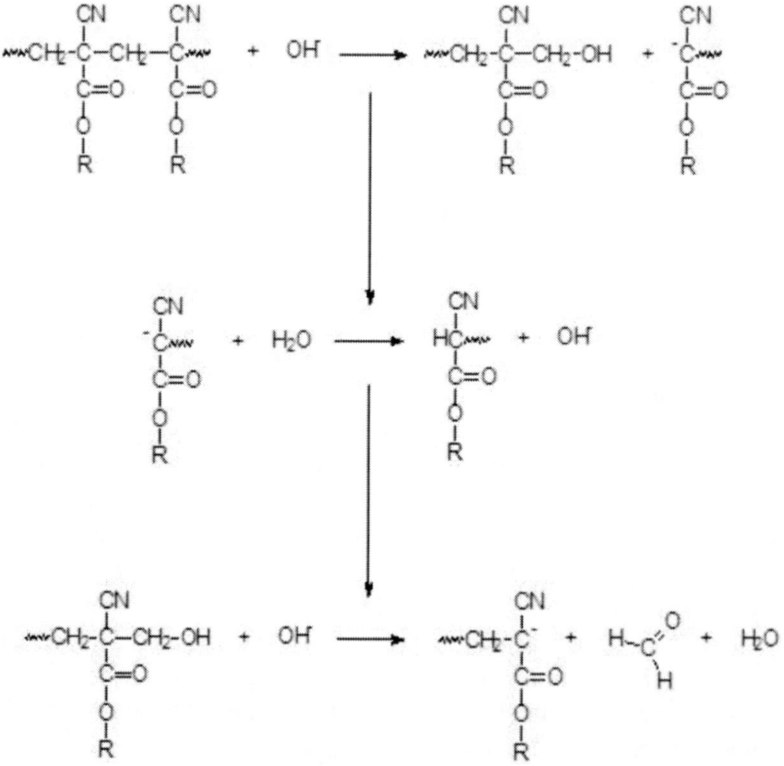

Figure 3. Methyl 2-cyanoacrylate degradation in aqueous medium (Adapted from Kopecek and Ulbrich, 1983).

This toxicity is a result of the degradation of cyanoacrylates in an aqueous medium into an alkyl cyanoacetate and formaldehyde (Kopecek e Ulbrich, 1983), (Figure 3). The resultant formaldehyde is the main responsible for the toxicological effects of these materials.

Table 2. Cyanoacrylate degradation rate

Alkyl group	% Degradation
Methyl	52,2
Ethyl	3,10
Propyl	1,99
Isobutyl	1,52
Butyl	0,73

As mentioned, the toxicity of cyanoacrylates is related with their degradation, or in other words with the release rate of their degradation products. Once again, the size of the cyanoacrylate alkyl group is the key for their toxicological profile. As shown in Table II, larger alkyl groups lead to slower degradation percentages and consequently, less toxic is the correspondent cyanoacrylate and therefore the adhesive (Park et al., 2002).

Besides the cyanoacrylates toxicity, other disadvantages to the use of these glues have been reported. They are responsible for inflammatory responses, allergic reactions, neural toxicity and also mutagenicity (Rietveld et al., 1981).For these reasons, the original cyanoacrylate formula discovered by Eastman Kodak (based on methyl and ethyl cyanoacrylate) was not approved by the FDA (Food and Drug Administration). Only in 1998, the FDA approved 2-octyl cyanoacrylate to be used in closing wounds and surgical incisions. Despite all of these facts, cyanoacrylates have been widely used in adhesion and to repair tissues (Handschel et al., 2006), blood vessels (Maldonado et al., 2003), lacerations (Howell et al., 1995; Mattick, 2002), plastic surgery (Silvestri et al., 2006) and in ophthalmology (Duffy et al., 2005; Setlik et al., 2005; Sharma et al., 2003).

Nowadays, cyanoacrylates are commonly used to treat minor lacerations due to their high strength and durability as well as due to their waterproof properties, which eliminate the need for wound dressing. However, their toxicity and carcinogenic potential restrict their use to external and temporary applications. FDA approved some cyanoacrylates to be available for medical application such as superficial wound closure, dermatology, and plastic surgery. They are commercially available under the brands Dermabond[TM], Soothe-N-Seal[TM] and Band-Aid Liquid Adhesive Bandage[TM] (Ryou, 2006).

2.1.2. Polyurethane Based Adhesives

Polyurethanes are one of the most versatile families of polymers. They can be prepared from a wide variety of materials exhibiting extremely different properties and therefore, a high variety of applications. This wide range of properties has attracted the attention of biomedical devices developers. They have been testing these polymers in several biomedical fields including pacemaker lead insulation, breast implants, heart valves, vascular prostheses and bioadhesives (Alves, 2012).

Urethane-based adhesives have been considered to be quite promising to be used as bioadhesives. Polyurethanes have characteristics that allow them to be considered as strong candidates to be used *in situ*, such as:high wettability properties with the majority of substrates; interact with the substrate by polar interactions (hydrogen bonds); ability to covalent bond with substrates with hydrogen atoms (when urethane pre-polymers are used) and by tailoring the molecular composition, the crosslinking degree and stiffness, urethanes can be moulded according to the desired application.

Polyurethane pre-polymers were first used as biological adhesives in 1959 for the fusion of bone fragments (Heiss et al., 2006). This adhesive, commercially named as *Ostamer*®, was composed by a pre-polymer and a catalyst which were mixed priory to application. However, the crosslinking reaction lasted 25 to 30 minutes and the adhesive showed to reach its maximal strength after 1 or 2 days. For these reasons, the experimental and clinical results revealed to be inadequate.

Since then, the development of urethane pre-polymers to be applied as bioadhesives as been an issue studied by different author (Lipatova, 1986; Sheikh et al., 2001; Ferreira, 2008), unfortunately despite the good adhesion results, the curing time is too long to face surgical demands.

From all studied polyurethane based adhesive studied, the most developed was KL-3 (Lipatova, 1986). KL-3 is a mixture of an excess of toluylene diisocyanate prepolymer (TDI, a mixture of isomers 2,4 and 2,6) with polyoxypropylene glycol and an accelerator of curing, dimethyltri (aminomethyl) phenol. The amount of accelerator predetermines the curing time.

Thus, the surgeon can adjust the curing time depending on the surgical situation. The adhesive cures under conditions of a moist area (since it is applied on the surface of an open wound) and presents the chemical structure presented in Figure 4.

Along the polymerization process, the reaction with water (present in the moisture of the wound) formed urea groups and released carbon dioxide. This causes foaming and the formation of a fine porous structure in the application surface.However the ability of adhesion of this material was evaluated and proved to be similar to cyanoacrylates.

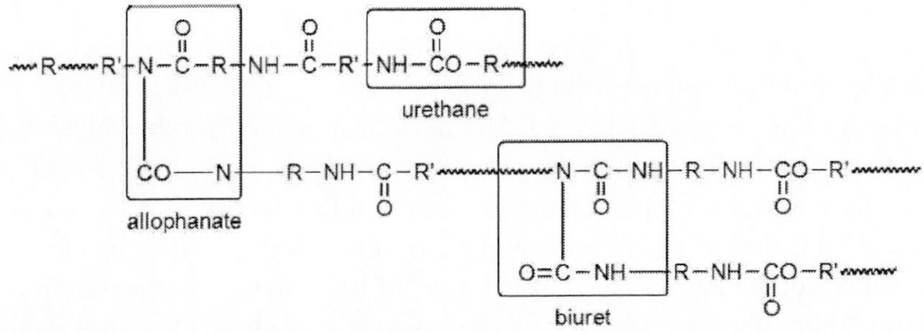

Figure 4. Chemical structure of the polymer network after curing.

The degradation was also evaluated and showed to be a hydrolysis process followed by elimination of the adhesive fragments by macrophages incorporation. This adhesive continued to be studied and was tested in several organs, such as kidneys (Nosov e Poliakov, 1980), endocrine tissue (Komissarenko et al., 1985), duodenum (Zemskov et al., 1985), pancreatic ducts occlusion (Zemskov et al., 1986), varicose veins treatment (Polous et al., 1996) and in hepatic tissue (Titarenko et al., 1994). However, these materials have been associated with local inflammation, cytotoxicity, and poor biocompatibility.Ultraviolet (UV) curable adhesives offer major advantages compared to pre-polymers systems, such as fast-curing rate, control of the polymerization heat evolution and are ideal for application to weakened and diseased tissue (Benson, 2002). Kao et al. (1997) have prepared UV irradiation curable bioadhesives based on N-vinylpyrrolidone. Although these adhesives presented suitable adhesive strength, the UV induced setting time was approximately 3 minutes, which is a value that should be improved when surgical applications are concerned.Ferreira et al. (2008) report the synthesis of urethanes based on polycaprolactone diol (PCL) easily crosslinked via UV irradiation to be used as a photocrosslinkable biodegradable bioadhesive. PCL is a semi-crystalline linear biodegradable aliphatic polyester that has been used in several medical applications already approved by the US Food and Drug Administration. Its structure presents several aliphatic ester linkages that can undergo hydrolysis and its products of degradation are either metabolized by being included in the tricarboxylic acid cycle or eliminated by renal secretion. The authors (Ferreira, 2008) modified the polymer with 2-isocyanatoethylmethacrylate (IEMA) to form a macromer that was crosslinked via UV irradiation using Irgacure® 2959 by CIBA as the photoinitiating agent. Results showed that after 60 seconds of irradiation the curing of the polymer was complete and membranes were obtained. The resultant films were then characterized by several techniques that included swelling evaluation, thermal characterization, surface energy determination, electronic microscopy, biodegradation in human plasma and haemocompatibility (haemolysis and thrombogenicity). In a global appreciation, it was concluded that the obtained membranes presented a porous morphology and that biodegradation occurred although in a slow rate (10% of weight loss after 6 weeks). Also, the material was haemocompatible (no significant value of haemolysis was measured) and presented thrombogenic character (which would contribute to control wound bleeding).

Finally, the adhesive was also able to promote efficient adhesion between the aminated substrates (gelatin was used as a model material), since during the binding strength tests the gelatin pieces broke without compromising the glued section. The adhesive was posteriorly tested in vivo using Wistar rats, in two organs (skin and liver) and it proved to be efficient in keeping the glued surfaces together (even in moisture conditions) for the entire experimental protocol. After this period the animals were euthanized and histological study of these organs was performed (hematoxylin and eosin coloration technique). No signs of necrosis or inflammation were detected in any of the target organs (Figure 5) (Ferreira et al., 2011).

2.1.3. Polyethylene Glycol Hydrogels

Polyethylene glycol (PEG) is a polymer with a simple structure (Figure 6) formed by two hydrogenated carbons, ether bonds and terminal hydroxyl groups.

PEG is soluble not only in organic solvents but also in aqueous solutions (Krsko et al., 2005), which makes it a good candidate for physiological systems. For molecular weights above 1000, PEG is also rapidly eliminated from the human body by renal excretion.

Moreover, PEG has the ability to imprint its characteristics when covalently linked to other molecules. Meaning that a toxic molecule can become non-toxic or hydrophobic molecular can became soluble in aqueous solvents when liked to PEG (Peppas et al., 1999).

Besides the previous advantages mentioned for PEG, other properties such as non-toxicity, biocompatibility and the ability to avoid immune system recognition (Corneillie et al., 1998) make PEG an excellent polymer to be used in the medical field. Moreover, for the same reasons PEG was allowed to be part of the strict list of materials approved by FDA for several applications, including biomedical applications (Popat et al., 2004).

PEG has been used in the development of controlled delivery systems of drugs (Ludwig, 2005, Serra et al., 2006), proteins (Van Dijkhui-zen-Radersma et al., 2005) and in the production of pro-drugs (Khandare, 2006).

In the tissue engineering field, PEG has been used for the preparation of release systems of growth factors for bone tissue in order to improve bone healing (Luginbuehl, 2004). In the area of tissue engineering, several authors showed that PEG hydrogels were suitable to be used as substrate of smooth muscle cells (Moffat et al., 2004); and PEG scaffolds were also good candidates for bone tissue cells for bone regeneration (Elisseeff et al., 2000, Martin, 2007).

In the particular filed of wound healing, PEG can be seen as a sealant, in other words, as a suture adjuvant that helps haemostasis in the wound. Nowadays, this kind of product is commercialized under the brands FocalSeal™- (Genyzme Biosurgery, Inc., Cambridge), CoSeal™ (Cohesion Technologies, Deerfield, IL) and DuralSeal™ (Confluent Surgical, Inc), among others.FocalSeal-L™ is a FDA approved photopolymerized hydrogel (Torchiana, 2003).

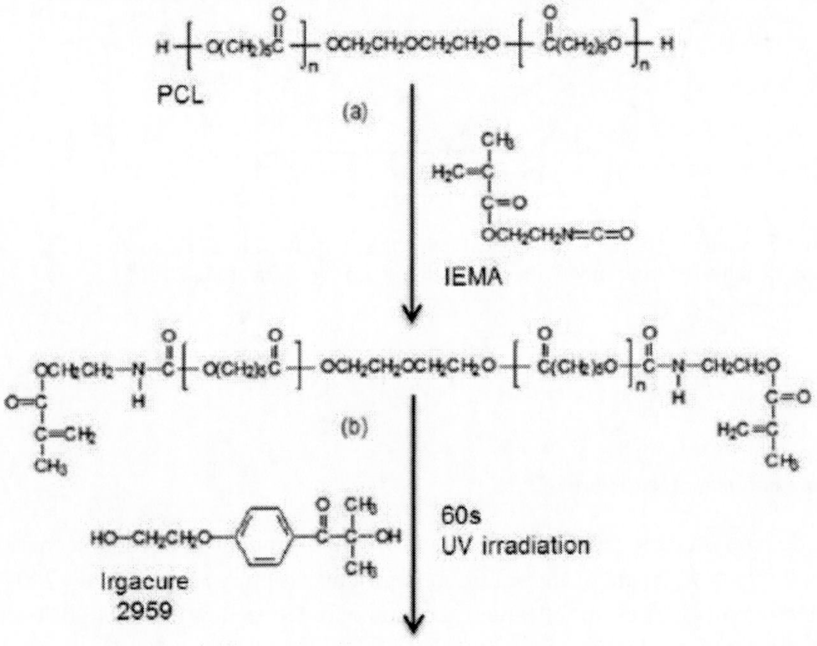

Figure 5. (Continued).

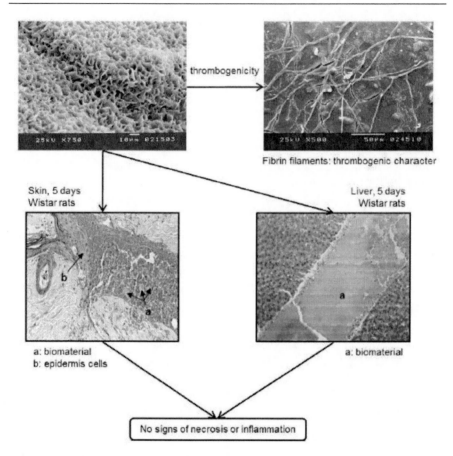

Figure 5. Summary of the development and characterization of a UV curable PCL based bioadhesive (reprinted with permission from (Ferreira et al., 2011).

Figure 6. Chemical structure of PEG.

Several studies express the efficiency of the product in several scenarios like: the reinforcement of the suture in ventricular ruptures (Fasol et al., 2004), protection of sutures in intestinal anastomosis (Sweeney et al., 2002) and prevention of air leaks from lungs in cardiac reoperations (Gillinov et al., 2001). FocalSeal-L[TM] was also tested in controlled release of oligonucleotides in mice, with the intent of used it in genetic therapy (Ramakumar, 2005).

For this propose, mouse model of partial nephrectomy were tested and PEG hydrogels revealed to provide adequate protection against renal hematoma and intraperitoneal blood, good haemostasis were obtained and oligonucleotides were carried throughout the kidney. Despite the good results, the time taken to prepare and apply the hydrogel is an issue, considering the need of a previous primer application, which limits the use when haemostasis is the priority.

CoSeal^{TM} other commercial available PEG product does not need photoactivation. This product is also used in surgery as sealant, mainly in vascular surgery (Wallace et al., 2001).DuraSeal^{TM} is used in neurosurgery as an adjunct to sutured dural repair during cranial surgery, in order to prevent the leakage of cerebrospinal fluid in the incision site. This product is composed of two solutions, a PEG solution and a trilysine amine solution. When mixed a gel is formed. The human body reabsorbs this gel within 4 to 8 weeks, allowing time for healing (Preul et al., 2006).

2.2. Natural Adhesives

Natural polymers, like some proteins (collagen and its derivatives, fibrin and even biomimetic mussels monomer like 1-3,4-dihydroxylphenylalanine (DOPA)) and some polysaccharides(like chitosan, starch and dextran) have so far been developed to be used as surgical adhesives. However, when it comes to commercial products, protein based materials are the ones more commonly used. The main advantage of protein based products, like collagen or fibrin glues is their intrinsic haemostatic properties that help in the coagulation process (Busuttil, 2003). For many years, these materials have been used as general-purpose glues, but due to their performance limitations they have been occasionally replaced by synthetic alternatives. However, they are still widely used as haemostatic agents, being sometimes combined with traditional wound closure methods such as sutures.

In 1838, Jöns J. Berzelins established the word "protein" to point out the importance of this class of molecules. The word comes from the Greek word *proteios*, which means "first class" or "first importance" (Nicholson, 2006).

Proteins like gelatin and casein have been widely used as adhesives for several centuries (Harrison et al., 2005). But, along the last decades, they have been replaced by synthetic polymers. Some of the proteins disadvantages are microbial and water sensibility as well as the relatively high price. However, the need to use materials from renewable sources have increased in the present days, therefore new applications for the, at the time, so-called "waste proteins" have been growing. This is the case of the proteins from the milk serum, which is increasing every day due to the increase of cheese and milk production. The use of this by-product to extract proteins and use them as adhesives would bring an increased value to the food industry.

In their native form, proteins have a globular or fibrous structure. They usually have regular structures such as α-helices or β sheet and turns, which leads to a very compact structure and to an internal density of about 75%. This might be a problem for the application of proteins as adhesives. An adhesive should be composed by long, flexible and crossed polymeric chains. With this structure, when the adhesive is exposed to a force to separate the adhesion connection, the formed network disperses the generated stress along the polymer bulk, not compromising the surface and protecting the adhesion focal point. Among the several proteins used as surgical adhesives, fibrin and gelatin are the most used since they show the previous optimal characteristic. Also, new approaches are being tested in order to develop new protein-based adhesives by recombinant DNA technique.

2.2.1. Fibrin

The use of fibrins as adhesives emerged, like cyanoacrylates, during the 50s, although they were used as a hemostatic agent since the early twentieth century. The first clinical use of an emulsion of fibrin in treating a wound date 1909 (Jackson, 2001). The fibrin is derived from blood clotting agents, in particular fibrinogen, factor XIII and thrombin. In its constitution still entersan antifibrinolytic agent (aprotinin) and calcium chloride (Ryou and Thompson, 2006). This material has a strong affinity for collagen, thus adhering easily to body tissues, in a case in which "mimic" the last step of the process of blood clotting (Petersen et al., 2004) (Figure 1-13). In the presence of calcium ions, fibrinogen and factor XIII is activated by thrombin, leading to conversion of fibrinogen to fibrin. The fibrin molecules polymerize to form a fibrin clot which is stabilized and strengthened by activated factor XIII (Figure 7).

Factor XIII is an enzyme(a transglutaminase) that catalyses the formation of covalent bonds between the side chains of different fibrin molecules, contributing to the crosslinking and rendering the hability of resisting dissolution (Ariens et al., 2002). The resultant bonds are peptide bonds formed between glutamine and lysineside chains resulting from atransamidation reaction (Figure 8). The transglutaminases have, for this reason, been classified as "nature's biological glues" (Griffin et al., 2002).

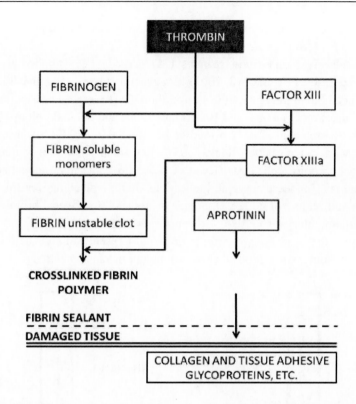

Figure 7. Simplified representation of the action mechanism of a fibrin sealant. The constituents of the sealant interact, when mixed, to form a stable fibrin clot that binds to damaged tissue. (Adapted from Dunn and Goa, 1999).

Furthermore, Factor XIII takes part in collagen synthesis by stimulating the proliferation of fibroblasts, contributing to wound healing. Additionally, aprotinin has the function of reducing the speed of fibrinolytic degradation of fibrin sealant, thus preventing its premature degradation (Spotnitz et al., 2005).

There are several physical and chemical processes used for obtaining the fibrinogen necessary to prepare fibrin glues and sealants, including cryoprecipitation and precipitation with ammonium sulfate, ethanol or polyethylene glycol (PEG). Cryoprecipitation involves several cycles of freezing/unfreezing and although being a time consuming process, it presents the advantage of not requiring the addition of exogenous chemicals (Silver et al., 1995). However, relatively low concentrations of fibrinogen are obtained by this method, which clearly reduces the effectiveness of the adhesive obtained. In contrast, chemical precipitation is a fast and efficient method to obtain high fibrinogen concentrations, but the purity of the final product is not, by any means, the desirable (Valbonesi, 2006).

The adhesives and fibrin sealants have already been applied in many surgical specialties (Morikawa, 2001) like general surgery (Sentovich, 2003), maxillofacial (Giannini et al., 2004) cardiothoracic (Kjaergard and Fairbrother, 1996), neurosurgery (Alibai and Bakhtazad, 1999) and ophthalmology (Yeh et al., 2006; Sharma et al., 2003), obstetrics (Contino et al., 2004), reconstructive surgery (Morris et al., 2006; Block, 2005). They are also commonly applied in several endoscopic procedures (Ryou et al., 2006). The main advantages of such materials for these surgical applications include bleeding control, tissue adhesion and sealing of defects in organs or tissues. Moreover, fibrin does not trigger inflammatory response or tissue necrosis (Morikawa, 2001).

Despite these advantages, fibrin does not present suitable hardness or stiffness for some applications that require higher mechanical strength.

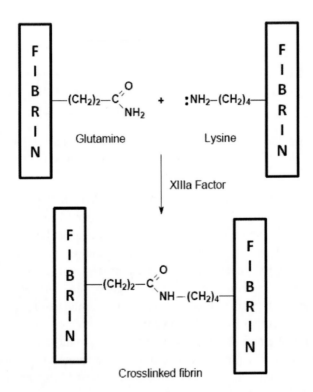

Figure 8. Fibrin is crosslinked by transamidation. Peptide linkages are formed between glutamine and lysine side chains.

Another drawback of this material is the risk of blood transmission of diseases. In fact, the use of fibrin sealants was banned by the FDA in 1978 because of the risk of viral infections transmission, particularly hepatitis B (Dresdale et al., 1985). Nowadays, with the increasing number of Acquired Immunodeficiency Syndrome (AIDS) and Bovine Spongiform Encephalopathy (BSE) reported cases new concerns arise regarding their application. One way of attempting to circumvent this problem is the extraction of fibrinogen from the patient's own blood (Dresdale et al., 1985). However, although this approach allows eliminating the risk of transmitting blood-borne diseases, it requires at least a two day preparation, and consequently a delay in surgery. Additionally, it is necessary to collect from the patient, approximately 1Unit of blood which may result in the need for a blood transfusion to replace the donated blood. However, this may be an impossible situation, depending on the patients' condition. For these reasons, the use of autologous fibrinogen is an impossible approach in situations of trauma, and emergency surgeries.

2.2.2. Gelatin

Gelatin is a derivative of collagen, which is a biodegradable polymer, soluble in water, with some industrial, pharmaceutical and biomedical applications. This material has already been applied in the preparation of microspheres used for the delivery of several drugs (Brime et al., 2000; Dinarvand et al., 2005) and in the production of biodegradable hydrogels (especially for burn treatment; Chang et al., 2003) and other controlled release systems (Yamamoto et al., 2003). Gelatin, although non-toxic, needs to be chemically modified with a crosslinker before it can be used as a bioadhesive. The primary purpose of this modification is to increase its adhesion strength and control its degradation rate.

The most common material used as adhesive, especially in cardiovascular surgery and surgery for aortic dissection, is a mixture of gelatin and resorcinol crosslinked with formaldehyde (usually named GRF glue). GRF was first used by Guilmet and colleagues (1979) and showed an improved survival rate for patients undergoing this type of surgery (Bachet et al., 1997). Although the application of this adhesive result in high strength bonding in tissues, its performance is restricted by the cytotoxicity associated with formaldehyde (Fukunaga et al., 1999). According to results reported by some authors, this could be the cause of many of the long term complications that arise in patients treated with this material (Kirsch et al., 2002; Tsukui et al., 2001). More recently, this compound has been replaced by another crosslinking agent: glutaraldehyde. Glutaraldehyde can be found in the composition of both gelatin and albumin adhesives, but, as in the case of formaldehyde, is associated with cytotoxic effects (Erasmi and Wohlschläger, 2002). For this reason, other crosslinking agents such as carbodiimides and genipin have already been tested *in vitro* (Sung et al., 1999; Liang et al., 2004).

Also, a new adhesive using a Schiff base reaction between the amine groups of modified gelatin and aldehyde groups introduced in polysaccharides (dextran and starch derivatives) by oxidation with sodium periodate (Mo et al., 2000). Their adhesive binding *capacity* was shown to be higher than the one of fibrin glue.

2.3. Production of New Protein Based Adhesives: The Recombinant DNA Technology

Although many proteins have been used as adhesives throughout history, the development of the recombinant DNA (deoxyribonucleic acid) technique presents new opportunities for the synthesis of proteinaceous materials. Additionally, many proteins traditionally obtained by extraction from animal tissues (eg, collagen, or mussel adhesive protein) are now being chemically or physically modified for novel applications in biotechnology and food industry (US Congress, 1993). In theory, proteins can be designed to present any structure and consequently, specific chemical and physical properties. The fact that one-dimensional genetic sequences may codify proteins with complex three-dimensional structures, confirms the power of nature in the synthesis of materials.

Some proteins which constitute a major structural material in various organisms have been extensively studied. Fibrous proteins such as collagen and silk have been the subject of considerable attention.

Other more specialized proteins like the adhesive protein responsible for binding bivalves (e.g. mussels) to rocks and ship hulls in the ocean are also attracting the attention of researchers.

A common feature to many of these proteins is the presence of repeated sequences of amino acids in their polymeric structure. These macromolecules or some of their specific regions, exhibit structural similarities with block copolymers.In the composition of the mussel adhesive protein, or more accurately the species *Mytilus edulis*, one of the most studied, there are actually five distinct proteins (Doraiswamy et al., 2006). All of them exhibit a block structure with repeating units similar to that shown in Figure 9.In the structure of these proteins, the DOPA (3,4-dihydroxy-L-phenylalanine) residues are responsible for the huge adhesive capacity of these proteins. The presence of phenolic groups allows the establishment of strong hydrogen bonding to various substrates and can also form chelates with metals.

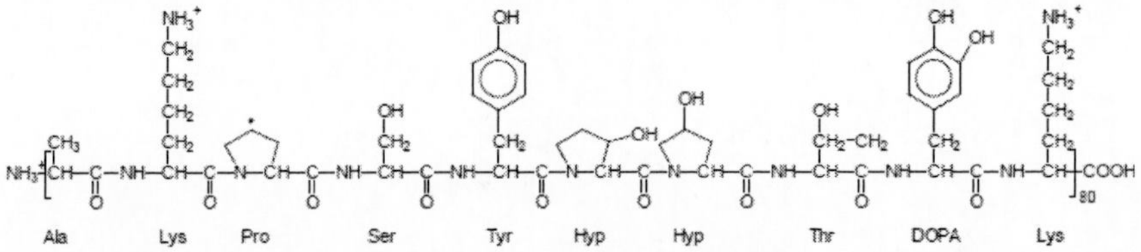

Figure 9. Repeating unit of the *Mytilus edulis* protein adhesive. Adapted from (Doraiswamy et al., 2006).

Some of these structural proteins were already chemically synthesized (Elmore, 2002). In this approach, specific peptides were created, which were then linked together to form a polypeptide (protein). However, chemical synthesis of proteins can be quite expensive and usually products lacking chemical and physical uniformity are obtained.

Conversely, the recombinant DNA technique allows the production of proteinaceous polymers with high purity, specific molecular weight and an excellent uniformity of characteristics.

These results are only possible because the exact sequences of amino acids in the proteins as well as the desired molecular weight are specified by the DNA sequence of the gene. For this reason, recombinant DNA technology may be an important strategy to prepare specific and high value materials that can be directly designed for a required application.

The major steps involved in recombinant protein production are shown in Figure 10. Several recombinant proteins are currently being produced (e.g. silk; Winkler et al., 1999) or investigated (eg, PAM, Hwang et al., 2004), using recombinant DNA technique. The fact that it is now possible to chemically synthesize genes containing the code for any repeating unit, gives almost unlimited possibilities of developing new proteinaceous polymers with unique physical and functional properties.

The early work on synthesis of artificial genes led to the creation of proteins that were able to be used as coatings, adhesives, membranes and medical or optical materials (Barron and Zuckermann, 1999).

CONCLUSION

Although the concept of gluing biological tissues can not be considered a novelty, the development of materials specifically designed for this purpose is in fact relatively recent.

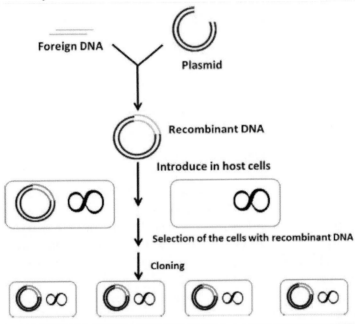

Figure 10. Construction and cloning of recombinant DNA molecules. (Adapted from Stryer, 1992).

Various materials presenting different chemical natures have been developed and tested to try solving some current surgical limitations. However, the variety of biological tissue requires the development of specific adhesives with precise properties making the task of obtaining products with multiple potential applications a very difficult one.

Indeed, it is important to understand that when it comes to surgical adhesives, it will be a challenge - or more likely impossible - to find a model that fits all uses ("one size fits all"), (Sierra and Saltz, 1996).

This is, and probably will continue to be the greatest challenge for those who which to do focuse their research in this intricate area that is as complex as interesting.

REFERENCES

Albala, D. M. (2003) Fibrin Sealants in Cardiovascular Surgery, *Cardiovas. Surg.* 11:5–11.

Alibai, E., Bakhtazad, A. (1999) Application of autologous fibrin glue in dural closure. *Irn. J. Med. Sci.* 24:92-97.

Alves, P., Ferreira, P. and Gil M.H. (2012) *Polyurethane: Properties, Structure and Applications: Biomedical Polyurethane-Based Materials* (1st ed). NY, US: Nova Science Publishers, Inc.

Ardis, A. (1949) E. Preparation of monomeric alkyl alpha-cyano-acrylates. *US Patent* 2 467 926.

Ariëns, R. A. S., Lai, T.-S., Weisel, J. W., Greenberg, C. S., Grant, P. J. (2002) Role of factor XIII in fibrin clot formation and effects of genetic polymorphisms. *Blood* 100:743-754.

Atta, H. M.; (1999) Edwin smith surgical papyrus: The oldest known surgical treatise. *Am. Surgeon* 65:1190-1192.

Bachet, J., Goudot, B., Dreyfus, G., et al. (1997) The proper use of glue: a 20-year experience with the GRF glue in acute aortic dissection. *J. Cardiac. Surg.* 12(2Suppl.):243-253.

Barron, A. E., Zuckermann, R. N. (1999) Bioinspired polymeric materials: in-between proteins and plastics. *Curr. Opin. Chem. Biol.* 3:681-687.

Benson, R.S., 2002. Use of radiation in biomaterials science. *Nucl. Instrum. Methods B* 191:752–757.

Block, J. E. (2005). Severe blood loss during spinalreconstructive procedures: The potential usefulness of topical hemostatic agents. *Med. Hypotheses* 65:617-621.

Brime, B., Ballesteros, M. P., Frutos, P. (2000) Preparation and in vitro characterization of gelatine microspheres containing Levodopa for nasal administration. *J. Microencapsul.* 17:777-784.

Busuttil, R. W. (2003) A comparison of antifibrinolytic agents used in hemostatic fibrin sealants. *J. Am. Coll. Surg.* 197:1021-1028.

Chang, W.-H., Chang, Y., Lai, P.-H., Sung,H.-W. (2003) A genipin-crosslinked gelatin membrane as wound-dressing material: in vitro and in vivo studies. J. Biomater. *Sci. Polymer Edn.* 14:481-495.

Contino, B., Armellino, F., Brokaj, L., Patroncini, S. (2004) Amniopatch, a repairing technique for premature rupture of amniotic membranes in second trimester. *Acta Biomed.* 75(1Suppl.): 27-30.

Corneillie, S., Lan, P. N., Schacht, E., Davies, M., Shard, A., Green, R., Denyer, S., Wassall, M., Whitfield, H., Choong, S. (1998) Polyethylene glycol-containing Polyurethanes for Biomedical Applications. *Polym. Int.* 46:251-259.

Dinarvand, R., Mahmoodi, S., Farboud, E., Salehi, M., Atyabi, F. (2005) Preparation of gelatin microspheres containing lactic acid – Effect of cross-linking on drug release. *Acta Pharm.* 55:57-67.

Doraiswamy, A., Narayan, R. J., Cristescu, R., Mihailescu, I. N., Chrisey, D. B. (2007) Laser processing of natural mussel adhesive protein thin films. *Mat. Sci. Eng.* C 27: 409–413.

Dresdale, A, Rose, E. A., Jeevanandam, V., Reemtsma, K., Bowman, F. O., Malm, J. R. (1985) Preparation of fibrin glue from single-donor fresh-frozen plasma. *Surgery* 97:750-755.

Duffy, M. T., Bloom, J. N., McNally-Heintzelman, K. M., Heintzelman, D. L., Soller, E. C. Hoffman, G. T. (2005) Sutureless Ophthalmic Surgery: A Scaffold-Enhanced Bioadhesive Technique. *J. AAPOS* 9:315-320.

Dunn, C. J., Goa, K. L. (1999) Fibrin sealant. A review of its use in surgery and endoscopy.*Drugs* 58:863-886.

Eaglstein, W. H., Sullivan, T. (2005) Cyanoacrylatesfor Skin Closure, *Dermatol. Clin.*23:193-198.

Elisseeff, J., McIntosh, W., Anseth, K., Riley, S., Ragan, P., Langer, R. (2000) Photoencapsulation of chondrocytes in poly(ethylene oxide)-based semi-interpenetrating networks. *J. Biomed. Mater. Res.* 51:164-171.

Elmore, D. T. (2002) Peptide Synthesis. In: Amino Acids, Peptides and Proteins, Ed. *The Royal Society of Chemistry*, Cap. 2, vol. 33, pp.83-134.

Erasmi, A. W.,Wohlschläger, C. (2002) Inflammatory Response After BioGlue Application. *Ann. Thorac. Surg.* 73:1020-1028.

Fasol, R., Wild, T., El Dsoki, S. (2004) Left Ventricular Rupture After Mitral Surgery: Repair by Patch and Sealing. *Ann. Thorac. Surg.* 77:1070-1072.

Ferreira, P., Coelho, J.F.J., Gil, M.H. (2007) Development of a new photocrosslinkable biodegradable bioadhesive. *Int. J. of Pharm.* 352: 172–181.

Ferreira, P., Coelho, J. F. J., Almeida, J. F., Gil, M. H. (2011). *Biomedical Engineering - Frontiers and Challenges: Photocrosslinkable Polymers for Biomedical Applications* (1st Edition). Reza Fazel-Rezai (Ed.), InTech Publisher.

Fukunaga, S., Karck, M., Harringer, W., et al. (1999) The use of gelatin-resorcin-formalin glue in acute aortic dissection type A. *Eur. J. Cardiothorac. Surg.* 15:564-570.

Giannini, G., Mauro, V., Agostino, T., Gianfranco, B. (2004) Use of autologousfibrin-platelet glue and bone fragments in maxillofacial surgery.*Transfus. Apher. Sci.* 30:139-144.

Gillinov, A. M., Lytle, B. W. (2001) A novel synthetic sealant to treat air leaks at cardiac reoperation. *J. Cardiac. Surg.* 16:255-257.

Griffin, M., Casadio, R., Bergamini, C. M. (2002) Transglutaminases : Nature's biological glues. *Biochem. J.*368(Pt2):377-396.

Guilmet, D. Bachet, J., Goudot, B.,Laurian, C., Gigou, F., Bical, O., Barbagelatta, M. (1979) Use of biological glue in acute aortic dissection.Preliminary clinical results with a new surgical technique.*J. Thorac. Cardiovasc. Surg.* 77:516-521.

Handschel, J. G. K., Depprich, R. A., Dirksen, D., Runte, C., Zimmermann, A., Ku☐bler, N. R. (2006) A prospective comparison of octyl-2-cyanoacrylate and suture in standardized facial wounds. *Int. J. Oral Maxillofac.Surg.* 35:318-323.

Harrison, S. M., Kaml, I., Prokoratova, V., Mazanek, M., Kenndler, E. (2005) Animal glues in mixtures of natural binding media used in artistic and historic objects: identification by capillary zone electrophoresis. *Anal. Bioanal. Chem.* 382:1520-1526.

Heiss, C., Kraus, R., Schluckebier, D., Stiller, A.-C., Wenisch, S., Schnettler, R. (2006) Bone Adhesives in Trauma and Orthopedic Surgery. *Eur. J. Trauma* 32:141-148.

Howell, J. M., Bresnahan, K. A., Stair, T. O., Dhindsa, H. S., Edwards, B. A. (1995) Comparison of Effects of Suture and Cyanoacrylate Tissue Adhesive on Bacterial Counts in Contaminated Lacerations. *Antimicrob. Agents Chemother.* 39:559-560.

Jackson, M. R. (2001) Fibrin sealants in surgical practice: An overview. *Am. J. Surg.* 182:1S–7S.

Kabanov, A., Okano, T. (2001) Challenges in Polymer Therapeutics, State of the Art and Prospects of Polymer Drugs: Polymer drugs in the clinical stage: advantages and prospects. New York: Kluwer Academic/ Plenum Publishers.

Kao, F.-J., Manivannan, G., Sawan, S.P., 1997. UV curable bio-adhesives: copolymers of N-vinyl pyrrolidone. *J. Biomed. Mater. Res.* 38:191–196.

Khandare, J., Minko, T. (2006) Polymer-drug conjugates: Progress in polymeric prodrugs. *Prog. Polym. Sci.* 31:359-397.

Kirsch, M., Ginat, M., Lecerf, L., Houë, R., Loisance, D. (2002) Aortic Wall Alterations After Use of Gelatin-Resorcinol-Formalin Glue.*Ann. Thorac. Surg.* 73:642-644.

Kjaergard, H. K., Fairbrother, J. E. (1996) Controlled clinical studies of fibrin sealant in cardiothoracic surgery - a review. *Eur. J. Cardio-Thorac.*10:727-733.

Komissarenko, I. V., Kebuladze, I. M., Lysenko, A. G., Shumova, T. V. (1985) Use of medical glues MK-6 and KL-3 in surgical endocrinology. *Klin. Khir.* 12:19-20.

Kopecek, J., Ulbrich, K. (1983) Biodegradation of Biomedical Polymers. *Progr. Polym. Sci.* 9:1-58.

Krsko, P., Libera, M. (2005) Biointeractive Hydrogels.*Materials Today* 8: 36-44.

Liang, H.-C., Chang, W.-H., Liang, H.-F., Lee, M.-H., Sung, H.-W. (2004) Crosslinking structures of gelatin hydrogels crosslinked with genipin or a water-soluble carbodiimide.*J. Appl. Polym. Sci.* 91:4017-4026.

Lipatova, T. E. (1986) Medical polymer adhesives.*Adv. Polym. Sci.* 79:65-93.

Ludwig, A. (2005) The use of mucoadhesive polymers in ocular drug delivery. *Adv. Drug Deliver. Rev.* 57:1595-1639.

Luginbuehl, V., Meinel, L., Merkle, H. P., Gander, B. (2004) Localized delivery of growth factors for bone repair. *Euro. J. Pharm. Biopharm.* 58:197-208.

Maldonado, T. S., Rosen, R. J., Rockman, C. B., Adelman, M. A., Bajakian, D., Jacobowitz, G. R., Riles, T. S., Lamparello, P. J. (2003) Initial successful management of type I endoleak after endovascular aortic aneurysm repair with n-butyl cyanoacrylate adhesive. *J. Vasc. Surg.* 38:664-670.

Martin, I., Miot, S., Barbero, A., Jakob, M., Wendt, D. (2007) Osteochondral tissue engineering.*J. Biomech.* 40:750–765.

Mattick, A. (2002) Use of tissue adhesives in the management of paediatric lacerations.*Emerg. Med. J.* 19:382-385.

Mo, X., Iwata, H., Matsuda, S., Ikada, Y. (2000) Soft tissue adhesive composed of modified gelatin and polysaccharides. *J. Biomater. Sci. Polym. Ed.* 11:341-351.

Moffat, K. L., Marra, K. G. (2004) Biodegradable Poly(ethylene glycol) Hydrogels Crosslinked with Genipin for Tissue Engineering Applications. *Appl. Biomater.* 71B: 181-187.

Morikawa, T. (2001) Tissue sealing.*Am. J. Surg.* 182:29S–35S.

Morris, M. S., Morey, A. F., Stackhouse, D. A., Santucci, R. A. (2006) Fibrin sealant as tissue glue: Preliminary experience in complex genitalreconstructive surgery. *Urology* 67:688-691.

Nicholson, J. W. (2006) Polymer Chemistry. In: *The Chemistry of Polymers*, RSC Publishing, UK, Cap. 1.

Nosov, A. T., Poliakov, A. A. (1980) Morphological characteristics of the renal tissue reaction to KL-3 polyurethane glue in kidney failure.*Klin. Khir.* 12:16-19.

Park, D. H., Kim, S. B., Ahn, K.-D., Kim, E. Y., Kim, Y. J., Han, D. K.(2002) In vitro degradation and cytotoxicity of alkyl 2-cyanoacrylate polymers for application to tissue adhesives. *J. Appl. Polym. Sci.* 89:3272-3278.

Patel, J. K. (2010). *Colloids in Biotechnology: Bioadhesive microspheres and their biothecnological and pharmaceutical applications* (1st ed). CRC Press: Taylor and Francis Group.

Peppas, N. A., Keys, K. B., Torres-Lugo, M. (1999) Poly(ethylene glycol)-containing hydrogels in drug delivery. *J. Control. Release* 62: 81–87.

Petersen, B., Barkun, A., Carpenter, S., Chotiprasidhi, P., Chuttani, R., Silverman, W., Hussain, N., Liu, J., Taitelbaum, G., Ginsberg, G. G. (2004) Tissue adhesives and fibrin glues. *Gastrointest. Endosc.* 60:327-333.

Polous, I. M., Hoshchyns'kyi, V. B., Chyzhyshyn, B. Z. (1996) The use of the polyurethane adhesive compound KL-3 for treating varicosities of the surface veins. *Klin. Khir.* 7:26-27.

Popat, K. C., Mor, G., Grimes, C., Desai, T. A. (2004) Poly (ethylene glycol) grafted nanoporous alumina membranes. *J. Membrane Sci.* 243:97-106.

PPTI: Protein Polymer Technologies, Inc. (2000) Sealing the market for Surgical Adhesives. *MedProMonth* 8:1-9.

Preul, M. C., Campbel, P. K. Bennett, S. L., Muench, T. R (2006) A Unique Dual-function Device – A Dural Sealant with Adhesion-prevention Properties.*European Musculoskeletal Review* 41-44.

Ramakumar, S., Phull, H., Purves, T., Funk, J., Copeland, D., Ulreich, J. B., Lai, L.-W., Lien, Y.-H. H. (2005) Novel delivery of oligonucleotides using a topical hydrogel tissue sealant in a murine partial nephrectomy model. *J. Urol.* 174:1133-1136.

Rietveld, E. C., Garnaat, M. A., Seutter-Berlage, F. (1981) Bacterial mutagenicity of some methyl 2-cyanoacrylates and methyl 2-cyano-3-phenylacrylates. *Mutat. Res.* 188:97–104.

Ryou, M. and Thompson, C.C. (2006) Tissue Adhesives: A Review. *Tech. Gastrointest. Endosc.*8:33-37.

Ryou, M., Thompson, C. C. (2006) Tissue Adhesives: A Review. *Tech. Gastrointest. Endosc.* 8:33-37.

Seewald, S., Sriram, P.V.J., Nagra, M. (2002) The expert approach: cyanoacrylate glue in gastric variceal bleeding. *Endoscopy* 34:926-932.

Sentovich, S. M. (2003) Fibrin Glue for Anal Fistulas: Long-Term Results. Dis. *Colon Rectum* 46:498-502.

Serra, L., Doménech, J., Peppas, N. A. (2006) Design of poly(ethylene glycol)-tethered copolymers as novel mucoadhesive drug delivery systems. *Eur. J. Pharm. Biopharm.* 63:11-18.

Serra, L., Doménech, J., Peppas, N. A. (2006) Design of poly(ethylene glycol)-tethered copolymers as novel mucoadhesive drug delivery systems. *Eur. J. Pharm. Biopharm.* 63:11-18.

Setlik, D. E., Seldomridge, D. L., Adelman, R. A., Semchyshyn, T. M., Afshari, N. A. (2005) The Effectiveness of Isobutyl Cyanoacrylate Tissue Adhesive for the Treatment of Corneal Perforations. *Am. J. Ophthalmol.* 140:920-921.

Sharma, A., Kaur, R., Kumar, S., Gupta, P., Pandav, S., Patnaik, B. Gupta, A. (2003) Fibrin glue versus N-butyl-2-cyanoacrylate in corneal perforations.*Ophthalmology* 110:291-298.

Sharma, A., Kaur, R., Kumar, S., Gupta, P., Pandav, S., Patnaik, B. Gupta, A. (2003) Fibrin glue versus N-butyl-2-cyanoacrylate in corneal perforations.*Ophthalmology* 110:291-298.

Sheikh, N., Katbab, A. A., Mirzadeh, H. (2000) Isocyanate-terminated urethane prepolymer as bioadhesive base material: synthesis and characterization. *Int. J. Adhes. Adhes.* 20:299-304.

Silver, F. H., Wang, M.-C., Pins, G. D. (1995) Preparation and use of fibrin glue in surgery. *Biomaterials* 16:891-903.

Silvestri, A., Brandi, C., Grimaldi, L., Nisi. G., Brafa. A., Calabrò, M., D'Aniello, C. (2006) Octyl-2-Cyanoacrylate Adhesive for Skin Closure and Prevention of Infection in Plastic Surgery. *Aesth. Plast. Surg.* 30:695-699.

Spotnitz, W. D., Burks, S. G., Prabhu, R. (2005) Fibrin-Based Adhesives and Hemostatic Agents. In: *Tissue Adhesives in Clinical Medicine*, Ed: James V. Quinn, B. C., Decker Inc., Cap. 4.

Stryer, L. (1995) *Exploring genes: Biochemistry*, W.H. Freeman and Company, Cap. 6, pp. 126.

Sung, H.-W.,Huang, D.-M., Chang, W.-H., Huang, R.-N., Hsu J.-C.(1999) Evaluation of gelatin hydrogel crosslinked with various crosslinking agents as bioadhesives: In vitro study. *J. Biomed. Mater. Res.* 46:520-530.

Sweeney, T., Rayan, S., Warren, H., Rattner, D. (2002) Intestinal anastomoses detected with a photopolymerized hydrogel. *Surgery* 131:185-189.

Titarenko, I. V., Pkhakadze, G. A., Galatenko, N. A., Savitskaia, E. S. (1994) Regeneration of the liver by using modified polymer compounds for the purpose of hemostasis. *Vestn. Khir. Im. Grekov.*152:17-23.

Torchiana, D. F. (2003) Polyethylene Glycol Based Synthetic Sealants: Potential Uses in Cardiac Surgery. *J. Cardiac. Surg.* 18:504-506.

Tsukui, H., Aomi, S., Nishida, H., Endo, M., Koyanagi, H., (2001) Ostial Stenosis of Coronary Arteries After Complete Replacement of Aortic Root Using Gelatin-Resorcinol-Formaldehyde Glue. *Ann. Thorac. Surg.* 72:1733-1735.

Valbonesi, M. (2006) Fibrin glues of human origin.*Best Pract. Res. Cl. Ha.*19:191-203.

Van Dijkhuizen-Radersma, R., Métairie, S., Roosma, J. R., De Groot, K., Bezemer, J. M. (2005) Controlled release of proteins from degradable poly(ether-ester) multiblock copolymers. *J. Control. Release* 101:175-186.

Wallace, D. G., Cruise, G. M., Rhee, W. M., Schroeder, J. A., Prior, J. J., Ju, J., Maroney, M., Duronio, J., Ngo, M. H., Estridge, T., Coker, G. C. (2001) A Tissue Sealant Based on Reactive Multifunctional Polyethylene Glycol. *J. Biomed. Mater. Res. (Appl. Biomater.)* 58:545–555.

Winkler, S., Szela, S., Avtges, P., Valluzzi, R., Kirschner, D. A., Kaplan, D. (1999) Designing recombinant spider silk proteins to control assembly.*Int. J. Biol. Macromol.* 24:265-270.

Woodward, S. C., Herrmann, J. B., Cameron, J. L., Brandes, G., Pulaski, E. J., Leonard, F. (1965) Histotoxicity of Cyanoacrylate Tissue Adhesive in the *Rat. Ann. Surg.* 162: 113-122.

Yamamoto, M., Takahashi, Y., Tabata, Y. (2003) Controlled release by biodegradable hydrogels enhances the ectopic bone formation of bone morphogenetic protein. *Biomaterials* 24:4375-4383.

Yeh, D. L., Bushley, D. M., Kim, T. (2006) Treatment of Traumatic LASIK Flap Dislocation and Epithelial Ingrowth With Fibrin Glue. *Am. J. Ophthalmol.* 141:960-962.

Zemskov, V. S., Biletskii, V. I., Panchenko, S. N., Shchitov, V. S., Blagodarov, V. N. (1986) Clinico-morphological characteristics of chronic pancreatitis in pancreatic duct occlusion using KL-3 glue. *Klin. Khir.* 11: 3-5.

Zemskov, V. S., Kolesnikov, E. B., Panchenko, S. N., Vozianov, S. A. (1985) Use of medical glue KL-3 in surgery of organs of the hepatopancreatoduodenal zone. *Khirurgiya* 61:37-39.

In: Recent Advances in Adhesions Research   ISBN: 978-1-62417-447-6
Editors: A. McFarland and M. Akins   © 2013 Nova Science Publishers, Inc.

Chapter 4

INTERACTION OF DIAMOND-TRANSITION METAL SUBSTRATES AND INTERFACIAL ADHESION ENHANCEMENT/FAILURE MECHANISM

Y. S. Li[1,2], Q. Yang[1] and A. Hirose[2]*

[1]Department of Mechanical Engineering,
University of Saskatchewan, Saskatoon, Canada
[2]Plasma Physics Laboratory, University of Saskatchewan,
Saskatoon, Canada

ABSTRACT

Diamond coating on the conventional transition metal substrates Cr, Fe, Co, Ni, Cu, Ti and their alloys is a promising technology for both structural and functional applications by providing enhanced surface wear/corrosion resistance or thermal conductivity. A major technical barrier so far is that complex interfacial reaction occurs between the gaseous precursors and the substrate components depending on the reactivity, solubility or diffusivity of carbon hydrogen and or oxygen with the metal elements. Especially, the Fe, Co, Ni are strong catalytic elements for preferential formation of non-diamond carbon phases on the

---

* Corresponding author: Y. S. Li. Department of Mechanical Engineering, University of Saskatchewan, Saskatoon SK S7N 5A9, Canada. E-mail: yuanshi_li@yahoo.com.

substrate surfaces, causing spontaneous spallation of the diamond films once they form. Cu and Ti have no such catalytic effects but mismatch in the thermal expansion coefficient with diamond exists, which also raises severe interfacial adhesion problems. We have performed comprehensive investigations on the diamond deposition on these typical transition metals in terms of nucleation, growth and interfacial bonds, and the adhesion issues are addressed by using high resolution TEM interfacial investigation and synchrotron radiation based analytical technologies. In this chapter, we will introduce our most recent progress in the understanding of diamond-substrate interaction and the mechanism of enhanced interfacial adhesion of diamond coatings on the related substrates.

1. INTRODUCTION

1.1. Properties of Diamond

Diamond is one of the most promising materials for advanced industrial applications such as in heat sink, optical devices, electronic devices, wear resistant protective coatings due to its extraordinary functions involving mechanical, physical, chemical and many other advantages [1]. Diamond is the hardest known material and has the highest bulk modulus and the lowest compressibility. It has the lowest coefficient of thermal expansion at room temperature and a high thermal conductivity. In addition, diamond is electrically insulating and optically transparent from deep ultra-violet to far infrared. Diamond is resistant to chemical corrosion and biologically compatible [2]. Given these unique properties, diamond has been regarded as a 21st-centrury high performance material and has a good prospect of application and extension.

1.2. Current Situation of Diamond Coating on Hetero-Substrates

Single crystalline, polycrystalline, nanocrystalline diamond films have been artificially synthesized at sub-atmospheric pressures on various hetero-substrates such as metal, ceramics, polymer, et al., by chemical vapor deposition (CVD) techniques. This novel processing technique provides an economically viable alternative to the traditional high temperature high pressure method, and has significantly extended application areas of diamond as protective or functional coating materials. Three classes of hetero-substrate materials can be sub-divided regarding the basic carbon-substrate interaction:

a   Little or no carbon solubility or reaction. These materials include such metals as Cu, Sn, Pb, Ag, and Au as well as non-metals Ge, sapphire, and graphite.

b   Carbide Formers. These include metals such as Ti, Zr, Hf, Si, V, Nb, Ta, Cr, Mo, Al, Mn, W, Fe, Co, Ni, Y and some other rare earth metals.

c   Significant C diffusion. In this case, the substrate acts as a carbon sink and the deposited carbon dissolves into the metal substrate and forms a solid solution or carbide. Such metals include Pt, Pd, Fe, Co, Ni, Mn and Ti.

CVD of diamond coatings on non-diamond substrates usually involves an initial formation of interfacial layer of carbide upon which the diamond subsequently grows [3]. Therefore, it is difficult to synthesize fast-growing and well adherent diamond thin films directly on those first class metals including Cu, Au, Ag, because of the lack of carbide formation between diamond and the metal surface. The second class metals among the above mentioned materials are considered to be favorable for rapid production of diamond film. Particularly, Si has been selected for long as a standard material due to its thermal and chemical compatibility to diamond which ensures adequate nucleation density, growth rates and adhesion ability of diamond thin films. Some researchers have confirmed that diamond nucleates and grows on the top of a SiC intermediate layer formed during the initial stage of the deposition process.

In addition, Si-containing compounds such as SiO_2, quartz, and Si_3N_4 also form carbide layers. For some metals like Ti and Cr, the TiC or CrxCy carbide layer grown at the early stage of diamond deposition can be several tens or even hundred μm thick [4, 5]. Such a thick interfacial carbide layer might significantly affect the mechanical properties, and the utility of CVD diamond coatings on these materials must be very careful. Substrates composed of carbides themselves, such as SiC, WC, TiC and Si_3N_4-SiC are particularly amenable to diamond deposition. The third class metals Fe, Co, Ni and their alloys and compounds like WC-Co, carbon steel, stainless steels, and tool steels, stand for the least successful substrates for deposition of adherent diamond films, which demonstrate slow nucleation rate, low nucleation density, and poor adhesion strength of diamond films. This chapter has primarily focused on our most recent achievements regarding successful coating of high quality diamond films on such ferrous-substrates, which has been once considered difficult or impossible.

2. DIAMOND COATINGS ON TRANSITION METALS

2.1. Benefits of Diamond Coatings on Transition Metals

In comparison with other substrate materials, steels are the most commonly used and cost-effective structural materials in many aspects of modern industry, and they have been widely applied as taps, dies, twist drills, reamers, saw blades, and cutting tools. The properties of steels can be greatly adjusted by designing the initial composition and optimizing the microstructures through subsequent thermo-mechanical treatment. Basically, when steels are used as critical components in harsh (wear, corrosive and erosive) environments, accelerated damage easily occurs.

As the early failure is usually initiated from the outer-most surface, it is important and cost-effective to obtain strengthened high performance surface for longevity of service.

It is a promising idea to deposit dense, continuous and well adherent diamond films on steels so as to obtain engineered surface properties, without deteriorating the strength and toughness of steel substrates. The duplex diamond/steel system will yield properties much superior to those of individual steel and diamond, allowing enhanced product performance and lifetime.

For instance, the diamond coated steel can possess increased surface hardness and anticorrosion behavior while retaining its tough core. Previous study indicated that a several microns thick diamond film could increase the surface hardness of steels up to 80 GPa and the lifetime of 304 SS was even increased by factors of several hundreds against high impact wear [1]. A one micron diamond coating also increased the resistance of steel to low impact wear from abrasives by a factor of 60. This represents significant increases in the life of the steel substrates.

In addition, the successful coating of high quality diamond thin film with controlled structures on steel substrates will provide cost-effective substitutes for cemented carbides and other hard tools for industrial applications, as well as prevent steels from humidity, abrasion, corrosion or other deformations in various industrial applications [6, 7].

2.2. Barriers for Diamond Coating on Transition Metals

Even though the CVD synthesis of diamond films on a range of substrate materials like silicon wafers and ceramics, has become very successful, CVD diamond on transition metal substrates (iron, cobalt, nickel) and these metal-based alloy steels is still a great challenge due to problems with nucleation and adhesion [8, 9]. The typical limiting factors making the direct nucleation, growth and good adhesion of diamond film on steel troublesome include:

a.   The Carbon atom has a high diffusion coefficient in Fe, Ni, Co or Mn matrix.

Metals such as tungsten, titanium, tantalum and zirconium react with carbon to produce carbides, while iron, cobalt, nickel and manganese dissolve carbon. As a result, under diamond growth conditions, deposited carbon dissolves into the steel matrix to form a solid solution, leading to a temporary decrease in the surface carbon concentration. Consequently, the onset of diamond nucleation is delayed due to the lack of a critical carbon supersaturation necessary for the diamond nucleation.

b.   Fe/Ni/Co acts as a catalyst for the formation of graphite.

Furthermore, carbon is too reactive with the Fe/Ni/Co elements and under diamond deposition conditions, these metals act as catalysts for the preferential formation of graphitic phase, which continues to remain as soot at the interface between the diamond film and steel substrates, leading to low nucleation rate/density and poor adhesion of diamond film on the steel substrate. The typical images are illustrated in Figure 1.

c.   The huge mismatch in the thermal expansion coefficients between transition metals and the diamond film.

Another major constraint in preventing the formation of continuous and adherent diamond films on steel is the large difference in their thermal expansion coefficients. The high elastic modulus of diamond leads to high thermal stresses during the process of heating up and cooling down, resulting in an increased tendency for crinkle, cracking, curliness and/or delamination of the diamond film. The large difference in the thermal expansion coefficient of diamond and steel also leads to very poor adhesion. As a combined consequence of the above detrimental factors, direct deposition of uniform and adherent diamond films on ferrous-base substrates without any special pretreatment has been scarcely reported [10].

3. TECHNICAL APPROACHES

Diamond deposition was conducted in a 2.45 GHz microwave plasma enhanced CVD system (Plasmionique) at a working pressure of 30 Torr. Both the substrate compositions and the plasma processing conditions were optimized to enhance the interfacial adhesion of diamond coatings on the substrate materials. A series of engineering alloys and home-made model substrate materials including pure Cr, Fe, Co, Cu, Ti, Fe-Cr, Fe-Ni-Cr, Fe-Cr-Al, Co-Al, Cu-Al, TiAl were used. These substrate materials selected have been prepared by melting the desired amounts of the component metals using an arc-furnace under Ar protection. The substrates were machined into specimens with dimension of 10 mm x 10 mm x 1 mm and polished with 600 grit SiC paper, cleaned in acetone and finally dried in a N_2 flow. The deposition was basically performed in a gas mixture of H_2 and 1 vol. % CH_4, while a much higher ratio of CH_4 gas was also applied for enhanced diamond nucleation. The microwave input power was kept at 800 and 600 W, producing a deposition temperature approximately 650 and 500 °C, respectively, as measured by a thermal couple mounted underneath the stainless steel substrate holder. The lowered deposition temperature is used to decrease the mismatch in the thermal expansion coefficients between the substrates and the top diamond coatings.

The general morphology, composition and structure of the diamond coating, coating-substrate interface and the underlying substrate were characterized by scanning electron microscopy (SEM), micro-Raman spectroscope, X-ray diffraction (XRD), atomic force microscope (AFM) and micro-hardness measurement. Synchrotron-based X-ray near-edge fine structure absorption spectroscopy (XAS), X-ray Laue micro-beam diffraction were performed at the 10ID-2, 06B1-1 and 07B2-1 beamlines of the Canadian Light Source, to address the bonding states of the diamond coatings and the structure changes (granular lattice orientation, coarsening, phase transformation) of the substrates.

Cross-sectional specimens for TEM observations were prepared by conventional method, i.e., by cutting, gluing, grinding with silicon carbide paper, dimpling to about 15 μm, and finally ion-milling by Ar^+ from both sides until perforation occurred. A SUPRA35 field emission scanning electron microscope (SEM) was used to observe the surface morphology of the films. A Tecnai G2 F20 transmission electron microscope was used at 200 kV for electron diffraction analysis, high-resolution transmission electron microscopy (HRTEM) observation. A Tecnai G2 F30 transmission electron microscope, equipped with X-ray energy-dispersive spectrometer (EDS) systems and a post-column Gatan imaging filter, was used at 300 kV for chemical composition analysis. The probe size for EDS line-scan was less than 2 nm and the step size about 3 nm. Energy-filtered images were performed using the three-window technique. To reduce the artifacts owing to the effects of specimen drift, the frame acquisition time was less than 30 s.

4. ADHESION ENHANCEMENT/FAILURE MECHANISM OF DIAMOND ON TRANSITION METALS

Our systematic research indicates that the diamond films grown on different transition metals show distinctive adhesion features depending on the substrate compositions and processing conditions.

4.1. Diamond Coating on Al Surface Modified Fe and Ni-Base Alloys

The early stage deposition of diamond on bare steel substrates has been extensively studied. A continuous diamond film can form on the steel substrate after a sufficient long period of deposition. However, this film in most cases spontaneously delaminates from the substrate after cooling down. After delamination of the top diamond layer from the substrate surface, a porous intermediate layer containing graphite particle and amorphous carbon is always observed. This non-diamond intermediate layer is primarily induced by the catalytic effect of the base metal Fe, Co or Ni and is responsible for the weak interface bonding between diamond coating and the substrate [2, 11].

In addition, a thick carburization zone in the substrate due to severe carbon diffusion is observed, as shown by an arrow in the cross-section image after delamination of the outer diamond film (Figure 1a). The corresponding XRD patterns (Figure 1b) indicate the presence of various carbides of iron and chromium, which are very detrimental to the mechanical properties of the substrates.

We have recently investigated the effect of surface modification of the conventional steel substrates by Al ion implantation or sputtering coating [12]. After ion beam implantation of Al, an Al-rich zone demonstrating a Gaussian like profile is present, and the implantation depth is calibrated to be close to 2 μm.

With increasing Al ion implantation dose up to 2×10^{17} ions/cm^2, the implantation depth is enhanced to 4.6 μm and the surface concentration of Al increases as well.

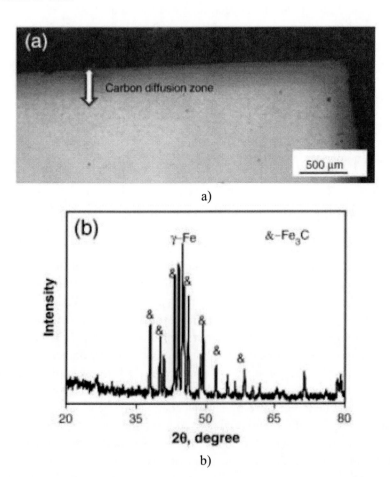

a)

b)

Figure 1. SEM cross sectional image of steel substrate after diamond deposition, (a) and the corresponding XRD patterns showing a significant carburization attack (b).

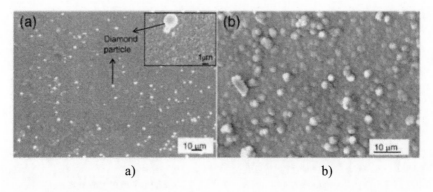

a)   b)

Figure 2. SEM images of diamond films grown on Al-implanted steels with different Al implantation doses. (a) A general view and a magnified view as insert for 5×10^{16} ions/cm^2 and (b) a general view for 2×10^{17} ions/cm^2.

Figure 1 shows the surface morphologies of diamond after 4 h deposition on steel substrates modified with different Al implantation doses. The deposition products formed on steel with a 5×10^{16} ions/cm^2 implantation dose of Al show a loosely packed composite structure consisting of sparsely distributed diamond particles, embedded in a matrix of graphite and amorphous carbon. In contrast, a continuous diamond film composed of spherical diamond particles has formed on the steel substrate implanted with a 2×10^{17} ions/cm^2 dose of Al. Each spherical particle actually contains more tiny diamond grains as revealed at a higher magnification.

Figure 3a shows Raman spectra of the top deposits formed on the Al-implanted steel substrates. With an implanted Al dose of 5×10^{16} ions/cm^2, a diamond characteristic peak centered at 1332 cm^{-1} of low intensity is observed, accompanied by a simultaneous presence of various sharp graphite-related peaks with much higher intensity.

This confirms that amorphous carbon and graphite containing a small amount of diamond has formed on this substrate. With an increasing Al implantation dose of 2×10^{17} ions/cm^2, the Raman spectrum of the spherical film shows a typical diamond peak but the intensity is low, and it has been incorporated into other non-diamond carbon peaks. Two accompanying peaks located at 1140 and 1470 cm^{-1}, respectively, are probably associated with nanocrystalline diamond phase or originate from trans-polyacetylene in the diamond film which still remains a controversial mystery.

However, more clear evidences are supporting that these peaks are related to hydrogenated carbon which are usually trapped in grain boundaries as well as on the film surfaces which increases with decreasing grain size.

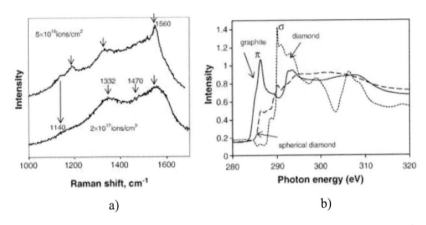

Figure 3. Raman (a, upper line is 5×10^{16} ions/cm^2, and lower line is 2×10^{17} ions/cm^2) and synchrotron XAS (b) spectra of diamond grown on Al-implanted steel substrate with a dose of 2×10^{17} ions/cm^2.

In addition, the graphitic carbon peak centered at 1570 cm^{-1} is broadened, and the peak intensity is significantly reduced in comparison with that formed with a low Al implantation dose. These SEM observation and Raman analysis demonstrate that an increasing Al implantation dose in the steel substrate can effectively enhance the diamond deposition, such as reduce the incubation stage to forma continuous diamond film. Normally, spherical diamond is more readily formed with higher CH$_4$ contents in the gas phase in order to increase carbon supersaturation, or by changing deposition parameters like plasma intensity and surface temperature. In this study, as the deposition is carried out at a relatively low methane concentration and under conventional deposition conditions, the formation of spherical diamond is most likely to be primarily effected by the substrate materials used. As described above, the base metals iron and nickel have strong catalytic ability for preferential formation of non-diamond, while the implanted Al is assumed to be effective to weaken this catalytic influence and supports the growth of diamond. As a consequence, the diamond deposition behavior on Al-modified steel substrates is closely dependent on the Al concentration, for instance, an Al implantation dose in this study. To more correctly characterize the bonding nature of the spherical diamond, synchrotron C k-edge NEXAFS spectrum recorded in total electron yield (TEY) is further used, as shown in Figure 3b. For comparison, typical graphite and diamond spectra are provided. The spectrum of diamond demonstrates a sharp absorption edge at 289.7 eV and a huge dip at 303.2 eV, corresponding to featured σ bonding of pure diamond. Graphitic carbon usually shows a sharp peak at 285.8 eV associated with sp2 structured π bonding. It can be seen that the major peaks of spherical diamond in the spectrum are located between those of diamond and graphite, indicating that the spherical diamond contains both p- and s-bonds.

Figure 4 shows diamond nucleation and growth on Al-interlayered steel substrates. After 20 min CVD deposition, diamond particles are sparsely observed on the steel surface and they appear to grow in certain direction following the scratches caused by SiC sandpaper treatment, while the uncovered substrate surface still remains clean and metallic luster (Figure 4a). The particle density increases with prolonged deposition time (Figure 4b, for 1.5 h). After 7 h, a dense, continuous diamond film is formed (Figure 4c). The diamond film shows a "cauliflower-like" surface morphology and no clear crystal faces are resolved. A fractured cross section observation of the diamond film reveals that the diamond film has a thickness of about 3.8 μm and it does not delaminate from the substrate, indicating that the diamond film has a good adherence to the substrate. It should be pointed that a thicker diamond film after longer time deposition is more easily subjected to local delamination from the substrate due to larger internal stress accumulated.

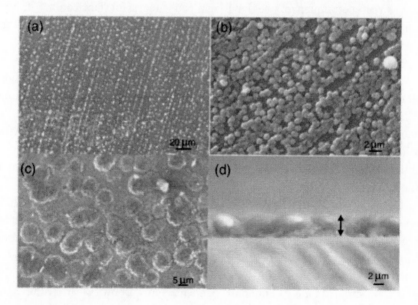

Figure 4. SEM images of diamond films grown on steel coated with an Al thin film followed vacuum annealing and diamond pre-scratching treatment. (a) 20 min; (b) 1.5 h; (c–d) 7 h.

4.2. Diamond Coating on Al-Bearing Fe and Ni-Base Substrates

Even though using an interlayer can in most cases solve the problem in obtaining high quality diamond film on steel substrate, this process is, unfortunately, relatively complex because multi-steps have to be applied to prepare intermediate layers which makes the diamond deposition complex and costly. Moreover, the interfacial adhesion strength at both substrate/interlayer and interlayer/diamond film has to be simultaneously guaranteed, which is sometimes especially critical for well-adherent diamond coatings on steel.

As an alternative approach, alternatives regarding a direct deposition of continuous and adherent diamond films on steel without using any external interlayers have been explored. This goal is likely to be achieved by modifying the steel using suitable alloying elements considering their different affinity with the reaction gases and diamond.

The related work on the direct fabrication of diamond films on various bulk steel substrates of different compositions revealed that the nucleation, growth, and adhesion properties of the diamond film are strongly dependent on the types and relative concentrations of alloy elements in the steel substrates. As a direct consequence, we have realized successful fabrication of high quality diamond films on specific steel substrates without using any interlayer or pretreatment [13-17].

Figure 5 shows typical SEM images of carbon deposits grown on Fe–Cr–Al substrates in an H_2-1% CH_4 gas mixture. The carbon films grown on them are quite different from those formed on Al-free steel substrates. A quick nucleation of diamond occurs on the Fe–Cr–Al steel substrate, and the uncovered steel surface around the diamond particles shows quite neat. After prolonged growth time, diamond micro-crystallites coalesce and form continuous and densely packed diamond film which also demonstrates a good adhesion to the substrate.

Figure 6 shows the surface morphology evolutions of diamond films grown on Fe–Cr–Al steel substrates when the substrate holder is further negatively biased with an induced glow discharge. Aligned diamond nanocones are even gradually fabricated on the substrate surface. Figure 6d is a top view of the cones with broken tips, indicating their solid cores. The Raman spectra of these diamond nanostructures show clear features of nanocrystalline diamond, for instance, the presence of a new pair of peaks at 1140 and 1480 cm^{-1} along with a significantly broadened diamond characteristic peak. The fraction of non-diamond phases such as graphite and amorphous carbon is assumed to be low.

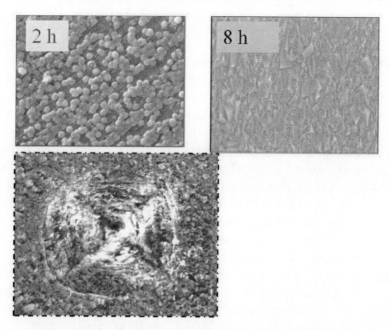

Figure 5. SEM images of carbon deposited for different time in an H_2-1%CH_4 mixture on Fe–Cr–Al substrate and an indentation test for adhesion evaluation.

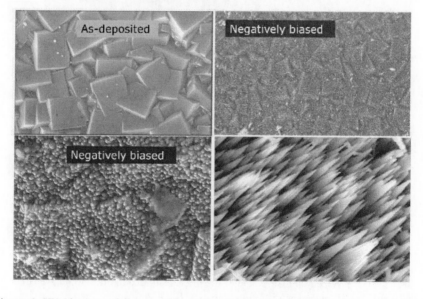

Figure 6. SEM images of diamond films deposited in an H_2-1%CH_4 mixture for 4 h on Fe–Cr–Al substrate, then continued on negatively biased substrate with glow discharge for additional (a, b) 20 min, and (c,d) 1 h.

Figure 7 shows the interfacial conditions of the diamond film prepared on Fe15Cr5Al substrate with 20 vol. % CH_4. Figure 6a is a low-magnification cross-sectional TEM image showing both the top ultra-fine diamond crystallites and the underlying FeCrAl substrate. A HRTEM image (Figure 7b) shows the details of this interface area indicated by a square in Figure 7a. The substrate is α-Fe in [100] axis. The nanocrystal diamond phase in the film is identified by an inter-planar spacing which is about 0.205 nm. Between the substrate and the film exists an amorphous interfacial layer, and the thickness of this layer is about 3-5 nm, which is much thinner than that formed with 1 vol. % CH_4. The composition of this interfacial layer shown in Figure 7c indicates that it is also an Al-rich layer. The counts of C and Fe were assumed to originate from the film and the substrate, respectively.

Energy-filtered transmission electron microscopy (EFTEM) is a parallel imaging technique, which gathers images from scattered electrons of a specific energy-loss range only. It can easily and quickly achieve a high spatial resolution at nanoscales. So this technique is very appropriate for investigating the elemental distribution in the narrow interfacial layer between FeCrAl substrate and diamond film.

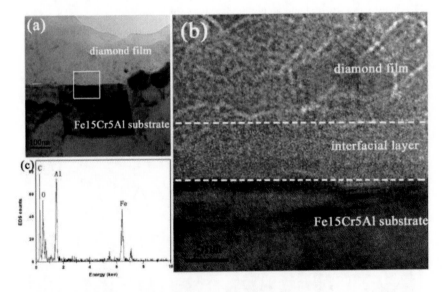

Figure 7. (a) Cross-sectional BF image of the interfacial area in the sample prepared with 20 vol. % CH_4 on Fe15Cr5Al substrate. (b) HRTEM image of the interface, the substrate is α-Fe along the [100] axis, an amorphous layer exist between the diamond film and the substrate; (c) an EDS point-scan profile scanned across the interface, showing the Al element concentration in the amorphous layer.

Figure 8a is the BF image filtered with zero loss peak (ZLP), where the interfacial layer shows a bright contrast. The corresponding energy-filtered mappings are shown in Figure 8b-e. The elemental spatial distribution is clearly visible by combining these mappings. The red dash lines indicate the boundaries of Fe (Figure 8b, substrate) and C (Figure 8c, film) maps.

A narrow interfacial layer exists between the two red dash lines. Figure 8d is the Al distribution map, while the red arrow denotes a layer where Al is enriched. The position of this layer is consistent with the narrow interfacial layer. Furthermore, a color mixed RGB image is shown in Figure 8f with Fe (green), Al (blue) and C (red). It clearly demonstrates that the interfacial area is an Al element enriched layer. In addition, the O element distribution (Figure 8e) is nearly the same as that of Al, revealing that, most probably, the Al element in this interfacial area exists in an oxide form. It is worth pointing out that the Cr element map is not included here because most of Cr element has formed carbides. It is interesting to note that in the case of a simultaneous presence of Cr and Al, many chromium carbide particles were observed to form at the interface between FeCrAl substrate and diamond film.

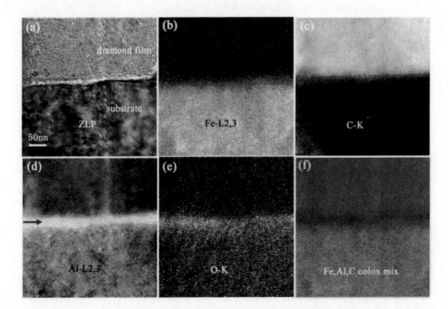

Figure 8. EFTEM images of FeCrAl/diamond interface demonstrating Al enrich in the interfacial layer. (a) BF image filtered with zero loss peak(ZLP); (b) Fe-L2,3 map; (c) C-K map; (d) Al-L2,3 map; (e) O-K map; (f) color mixed RGB image with Fe (green), Al (blue), C (red).

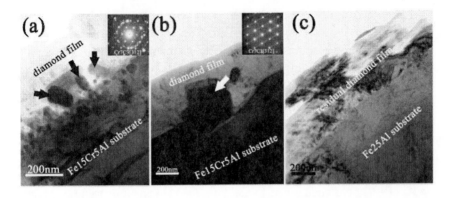

Figure 9. (a-b) BF images and corresponding EDPs of chromium carbides precipitated along FeCrAl/diamond interface; (c) BF image of FeAl/diamond interface, no carbide was observed.

Figure 9a-b shows the TEM images of chromium carbides precipitating at the FeCrAl/diamond interface, with the inserts showing the corresponding EDPs of the marked carbides. In some cases, the interfacial carbides are partially immerged in the substrate while the rest are incorporated into the diamond film.

4.3. Mechanism Proposed

Based on our analysis and discussion, a model regarding the Al and Cr alloying modification mechanism for diamond growth on Fe-base substrate is proposed, as shown in Figure 10:

a   On pure Fe substrate, the film consists of a loosely packed graphite intermediate layer and many iron carbide particles. A continuous iron carbide layer formed on the substrate surface.

b   Only single alloying by Cr, the film is the same as that on pure Fe substrate, and the difference is that large numbers of chromium and iron carbides form in FeCr alloy substrate, but no continuous iron carbide layer forms on the substrate surface, and the size of carbides are much smaller than that in pure Fe substrate.

c   Only single alloying by Al, the diamond film can form on FeAl substrate, due to the formation of an Al enriched interfacial layer. But the diamond film does not adhere well to the substrate and spalls locally.

d   Simultaneously alloying Al and Cr, diamond film not only can form on FeCrAl substrate, but also adheres well to the substrate. An Al enriched layer formed along the interface, furthermore, many chromium carbides precipitate at the interface and in the substrate.

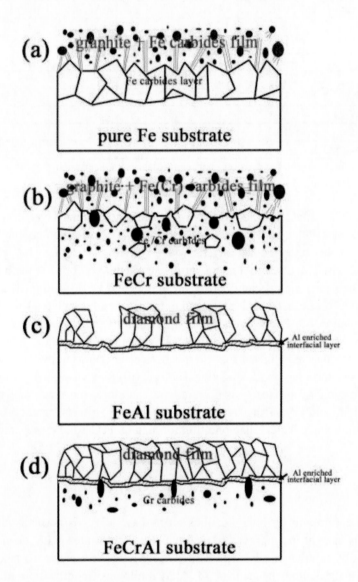

Figure 10. A simple model regarding the Al, Cr alloying modification mechanism for diamond growth on the Fe-base substrates.

Table 1. Thermal stress of diamond films on various substrates were estimated

	$\alpha\times10^{-6}$ [a]/K			σthermal
material	293K	943K	αAve	(GPa)
diamond	0.8	4.2	2.5	
Fe	11.8	16.5	14.2	~8.59
Cr	4.9	11.5	8.2	~4.18
Al	23.1	32.3(800K)	28	~18.7
Fe15Al	11.6	21	16.3	~10.13
Fe25Al				>>10.13
Fe15Cr	~10.5	~13.7	12.1	~7.04
Fe15Cr5Al				8.59>σ>7.04

[a]α is the linear thermal expansion coefficient (data from Thermophysical Properties of Matter, The TPRC Data Series).

In this model, it is necessary to point that a diamond layer may finally form on pure Fe or Fe-Cr substrate but it easily peels off upon cooling, due to the graphite intermediate layer, which is less meaning for practical applications. The role of Al is that an Al enriched layer forms at the interface, which acts as (i) an efficient barrier for both C and Fe diffusion; (ii) a crucial hindrance of Fe catalyzed preferential formation of graphite; (iii) a quick accumulation of C for supersaturation. Meanwhile, the role of Cr is to (i) reduce the Al concentration needed; (ii) enhance the interface adhesion as decreasing the thermal stresses and mechanical interlocking by the interfacial chromium carbides, as illustrated in Table 1; (iii) play an auxiliary role in the accumulation of surface C concentration. Therefore, the beneficial roles of element Al and Cr playing, especially the synergetic effects, promote a dense, continuous and adherent diamond film forming on FeCrAl alloy substrate.

CONCLUSION

Direct growth of diamond films on Fe-base alloys is normally difficult, but this has been improved by alloying the substrates with element Al, especially simultaneously with Cr. By our comprehensive cross-sectional TEM analysis, the mechanism of Al, Cr alloying modification effects is clarified. And a simple model regarding the Al, Cr alloying modified mechanism for diamond growth on Fe-base substrate is proposed.

A thin amorphous layer is observed to be formed at the interface between diamond film and FeCrAl substrate. According to the results of energy dispersive X-ray spectroscopy and energy-filtered imaging, this interfacial layer is especially rich in Al, along with a simultaneous O enrichment, so Al exists in the oxide form. The Al enriched interfacial layer acts as an effective barrier, which can hinder the diffusion of carbon species and suppress the formation of graphite on steel substrates, providing a stable surface for diamond nucleation and growth. In contrast, on pure Fe and FeCr alloy substrates, there are no efficient barrier to hinder the high diffusion of carbon and the graphitization effect catalyzed by iron, hence, the graphite phase has quickly formed at the interface and large numbers of carbides formed in the substrates.

In addition, in comparison with FeAl substrate, simultaneously alloying with Cr in FeCrAl substrate has three beneficial effects. First, the percentage of Al needed to develop a continuous protective scale is reduced. Second, the interface adhesion is enhanced between diamond film and FeCrAl substrate, which can be attributed to the decrease of substrate thermal-expansion coefficient by Cr added and mechanical interlocking by the interfacial chromium carbides. Finally, the chromium carbides precipitated along the defects in the FeCrAl substrate play an auxiliary role in hindering carbon diffusion.

ACKNOWLEDGMENTS

This study is sponsored by the Canada Research Chair Program and by the Natural Sciences and Engineering Research Council of Canada (NSERC). The synchrotron data were measured from the 10ID-2, 06B1-1 and 07B2-1 beamlines, the Canadian Light Source, which is supported by *the NSERC, NRC and the University of Saskatchewan.*

REFERENCES

[1]   May, P. W. *Phil. T. Roy. Soc. A.* 2000, 358, 473-495.
[2]   Xu, N. S., Huq, S. E. *Mater. Sci. engineer R.* 2005, 48, 47-189.
[3]   Jiang, X., Fryda, M., Jia, C. L. *Diamond Relat. Mater.* 2000, 9, 1640-1645.

[4]   Yan, B. B. *Surf. Coat. Technol.* 1999, 115, 256-265.
[5]   Ali, N., Fan, Q. H., Gracio, J., Ahmed, W. *Surf. Engineer.* 2002, 18, 260-264.
[6]   R. J. Narayan, *J. Adhes. Sci. Technol.* 2004, 18, 1339-1365.
[7]   Maguire, P. D., McLaughlin, J. A. *Diamond Relat. Mater.* 2005, 14, 1277-1288.
[8]   Chen, X., Narayan, J. *J. Appl. Phys.* 1993, 7, 4168-4173.
[9]   Spinnewyn, J., Nesladek, M., Asinari, C. *Diamond . Relat. Mater.* 1993, 2, 361-364.
[10] Davanloo, F., Park H., Collins, C. B. *J. Mater. Res.* 1996, 11, 2042-2050.
[11] Buijnsters, J. G., Shankar, P., Gopalakrishnan, P. *Thin Solid Films.* 2003, 426, 85-93.
[12] Li, Y. S., Ma, H. T., Yang, L., Yang, Q., Hirose, A. *Surf. Coat. Technol.* 2012, 207, 328-333.
[13] Li, Y. S., Hirose, A. *Chem. Phys. Lett.* 2006, 433, 150-153.
[14] Li, Y. S., Hirose, A. *J. Appl. Phys.* 2007, 101, Art. No. 073503.
[15] Li, Y. S., Pan, T. J., Tang, Y., Yang, Q., Hirose, A. *Diamond Relat. Mater.* 2011, 20, 187-190.
[16] Li, Y. S., Hirose, A. *Surf. Coat. Technol.* 2007, 202, 280-287.
[17] Li, Y. S., et al. Unpublished data.

In: Recent Advances in Adhesions Research   ISBN: 978-1-62417-447-6
Editors: A. McFarland and M. Akins   © 2013 Nova Science Publishers, Inc.

Chapter 5

INHIBITION OF CELL ADHESION: THE ROLE OF POLYSIALIC ACID IN THE INHIBITION OF CELL-CELL INTERACTIONS

Athanasios K. Petridis [*]

Wedau Kliniken Duisburg, Duisburg, Germany
University Schleswig-Holstein, Camous Kiel, Germany

ABSTRACT

Polysialic acid, an $\alpha2,8$-sialic acid polymer is specifically bound on the neural cell adhesion molecule (NCAM). PSA binds a significant amount of water molecules and serves as a spacer between cells, inhibiting trans- (NCAM-NCAM) as well as cis-interactions.

The PSA expression on neuronal stem cells prevents a premature differentiation of these cells through the inhibition of cell-cell adhesion signaling. Other interactions like integrin-$\beta1$ and NCAM on the cell membrane (cis-interaction) are ihnibited through PSA expression.

PSA expression on the surface of cells inhibits cell signaling and therefore this sialic acid polymer is responsible for inhibiting premature physiological changes of neuronal stem cells.

On the other hand it is also overexpressed on cancer cells, establishing the malignant cell phenotype of these cells. Cancer cell

[*] E-mail: opticdisc@aol.com.

interactions are ihnibited by PSA and therefore these cells do not interact with their environment and keep an „antisocial" state. By PSA overexpression cells do not bind with their environment and can migrate freely through tissues.

Stem cell migration is established, as well as migration of cancer cells rendering these cells highly invasive and metastatic.In the present chapter the mecahnism of cell adhesion inhibition through PSA is discussed.

INTRODUCTION

In the developmental stage of organogenesis of the CNS the $\alpha 2,8$-sialic acid polymer is overexpressed on the migrating neuronal pregenitor cells. This charged long linear homopolymer is attached to NCAM and through binding of water occupies a significant hydrated volume in the intercellular space acting as a down regulator of cell interactions (Fujimoto et al, 2001, Johnson et al, 2005). Quantitative biophysical experiments showed the hindrance of close conatcts between cells. The increased distance between cell membranes reduces cell-cell binding forces by inhibition of adhesion molecules like NCAM and Cadherins (Johnson et al, 2005). Through the reduction of cell interactions cell adhesion is inhibited and changes in organ structures can be created (Bruses et al, 2001, El Maarouf et al, 2006).

PSA is expressed on the surface of neural progenitors to prevent a premature differentiation of these cells and establish their migration through the rostral migratoty stream in the brain. After downregulation of PSA stem cells stop migrating, cell adhesion is established and differentiation starts (Petridis et al, 2004).

The inhibition of cell interactions is used by tumor cells establishing the de-differentiation of cancer cells and increasing the migratoty potential of these cells rendering their invasive and metastatic potential (Miyahara et al, 2001, Glüer et al, 1998, Petridis et al, 2009).

On the other hand, induction of PSA on the surface of reactive glial cells after lesion in the CNS changes the morphology of the glial scar and increases permeability of the scar for spinal cord axons through the scar (El Maarouf et al, 2006).

In the present work the function of PSA through global inhibition of cell adhesion in stem cells and in tumor cells will be emphasized. The overexpression of PSA on glial scars with change of the scar tissue morpholgy will be shown and discussed too.

PHYSIOLOGIC EXPRESSION OF PSA ON THE SURFACE OF NEURONAL STEM CELLS INHIBITS CELL ADHESION

PSA is expressed on the surface of neuronal stem cells in the subventricular zone (SVZ). These cells migrate through the rostral migratoty stream (RMS) to the olfactory bulb where PSA is downregulated and differentiation starts (Ono et al, 1994, Doetsch and Alvarez-Buylla, 1996, Hu, 1996).

The removal of PSA on the progenitor cells in the SVZ ex-vivo (explant cultures) and in vitro (intrathecal injections of endoneuramnidase N) with specific cleavage by endoneuraminidase N (endo N) inhibited cell migartion of SVZ cells in the RMS (Petridis et al, 2004, Ono et al, 1994). NCAM –deficient mice also showed inhibition of cell migration of neuronal progenitors since PSA could not expressed on the cells (Cremer et al, 1994).

Not only cell migration is inhibited. It could be shown that the inhibition of cell migration through removal of PSA had changed the morphology of the SVZ.

The progenitor cells changed their morphology and developed long neurites and expressed tyrosine hydroxylase (TH) mimicking the phenotype they would adopt in the olfactory bulb (Petridis et al, 2004). The cells started differentiating prematurely (Petridis et al, 2004). The cleavage of PSA in SVZ explant cultures showed also a premature differentiation of stem cells resulting in expression of βIII-tubulin and neurofilament-L in these cells showing their neuronal differentiation.

Removal of PSA from stem cells activates MAPK p44/42 through an NCAM / fyn pathway (Beggs et al, 1997). The activation of this pathway leads to differentiation (Petridis et al, 2004).

In explant cultures it could be shown that differentiation of stem cells through PSA-removal requiered cell-cell contact. PSA removal induced cell differentiation only in aggregates of more than 3 cells and did not show any effect in isolated cells.

NCAM has been shown to activate p59fyn and MAPK p44/42 phosphorylation and PSA inhibits the phosphorylation of these kinases (Beggs et al, 1997, Hoffman et al, 1998).

The removal of PSA induces cell adhesion and activates an NCAM induced differentiation (Petridis et al, 2004).

PSA EXPRESSION ON THE SURFACE OF TUMOR CELLS

PSA is overexpressed in highly invasive and metastatic tumors like small cell lung cancer, rhabdomyosarcomas, neuroblastomas and high grade astrocytomas (Glüer et al, 1998, Miyahara et al, 2001, Petridis et al, 2004, Suzuki et al, 2005, Petridis et al, 2009).

In a gain of function experiment, the PSA overexpression showed that glioma cells which express PSA increased their invasive potential (Suzuki et al, 2005). Since PSA is loosening cell-cell-interactions and decreases adhesive forces, it enables tumor tissue to become loose and tumor cells to leave the solid tumor tissue and invade in surrounding tissues or even metestasize.

In PSA expressing neuroblastoma cells (SH-SY5Y) the removal of PSA from these cells led to a differentiation of tumor cells only in cell aggregates showing that PSA removal allows cell-cell contact and activates NCAM-induced signaling pathways (Seidenfaden et al, 2003, Petridis et al, 2004). Additionally, the removal of PSA led to a more solid adhesive tumor tissue and inhibited cell migration in vitro (Seidenfaden et al, 2003, Petridis et al, 2004).

PSA OVEREXPRESSION ON GLIAL SCAR TISSUE OF THE SPINAL CORD ATTENUATES CELL ADHESION AND CHANGES TISSUE MORPHOLOGY

After lesioning of the adult mammalian spinal cord reactive astrocytes create an impermeable scar, which does not allow axonal growth through the scar tissue. The axons show an intrinsic ability to grow after lesion but the scar tissue is building a wall (Cajal, 1928, Batcholor and Howells, 2003).

It could be shown that axonal growth was observed in regions where a subpopulation of astrcytes in the scar tissue expressed PSA (Aubert et al, 1998, Dusart et al, 1999, Camand et al, 2004). PSA is known to alter glial cell-based architecture (Canger and Rutishauser, 2004).

The retroviraly induced overexpression of PSA on glial cells in spinal cord scar tissue led to decrease of glia-cell adhesion and allowed axons to grow significantly through the spinal cord scar tissue initiating regeneration (Petridis et al, 2006).

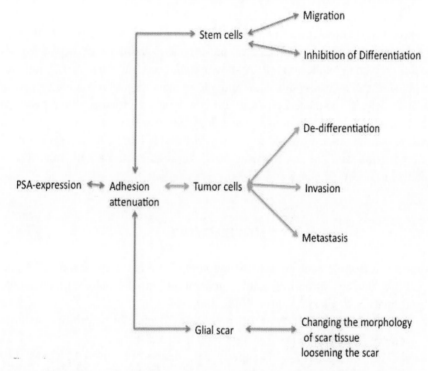

Figure 1. Regulation of Cell Adhesion through PSA. The chart shows the regulatory interactions of PSA and cell adhesion. The expression of PSA inhibits cell adhesion and leads to migration and the inhibition of differentiation in stem cells and invasion, de-differentiation and metastasis in tumor cells. A PSA overexpression in glial scar tissue changes the scar morphology and renders the scar permeable for axonal growth. The arrows are double ended to show that the effect can be amphidromal since a PSA downregulation leads to increased adhesion and opposite effects.

CONCLUSION

Cell adhesion is very important in the tissue forming process. It keeps tissue morphology intact. Never the less besides the adhesive forces there are regulators, which enable tissue plasticity. There are molecules that decrease adhesive forces between cells in tissues. This allows cells to leave the organ complex and migrate away from the „cell community". This effect is used from endogenous stem cells which need attenuated adhesion to migrate, as well as from tumor cells which leave the primary tumor to invade the neighbouring tissue and metastasize.

The attenuation of cell adhesion is enabled by polysialiac acid (PSA). PSA is expressed on the extracellular site of the cell membrane on NCAM. It binds a great amount of water molecules and increases the distance between cells decreasing their adhesion. PSA downregulation on the other hand re-establishes cell adhesion in tissues and allows activation of signaling pathways through cell-cell contact. Cell adhesion is a dynamic process, which needs to be regulated in both directions, up and down, to give tissues the opportunity to change their status from fixed to plastic. Molecules like PSA are regulators of cell adhesion and the mechanism how the regulation of cell adhesion is enabled has been emphasized in the present chapter.

REFERENCES

Aubert I, Ridet JL, Schachner M, Rougon G, Gage FH. Expression of L1 and PSA during sprouting and regeneration in the adult hippocampal formation. *J. Comp. Neurol.* 1998; 399:1-19.

Batcholor PE, Howells DW. CNS regeneration: clinical possibility or basic science fantasy? *J. Clin. Neurosci.* 2003; 10:523-534.

Beggs HE, Baragona SC, Hemperly JJ, Maness PF. 1997. NCAM 140 interacts with the focal adhesion kinase p125fak and the SRC-related tyrosine kinase p59fyn. *J. Biol. Chem.* 272:8310–8319.

Brusés JL, Rutishauser U. Roles, regulation, and mechanism of polysialic acid function during neural development. *Biochimie.* 2001; 83:635-43.

Cajal SG. *Degeneration and regeneration of the nervous system*, vol. 1 and 2. Oxford University Press, London.

Camand E, Morel MP, Faissner A, Sotelo C, Dusart I (2004) *Eur. J. Neurosci.* 20:1161–1176.

Canger AK, Rutishauser U. Alteration of neural tissue structure by expression of polysialic acid induced by viral delivery of PST polysialyltransferase. Glycobiology. 2004; 14:83-93.47.

Cremer H, Lange R, Christoph A, et al. Inactivation of the N-CAM gene in mice results in size reduction of the olfactory bulb and deficits in spatial learning. *Nature* 1994; 367:455-59.

Dusart I, Morel MP, Wehrlé R, Sotelo C. Late axonal sprouting of injured Purkinje cells and its temporal correlation with permissive changes in the glial scar. *J. Comp. Neurol.* 1999; 408:399-418.

Doetsch F, Alvarez-Buylla A. Network of tangential pathways for neuronal migration in adult mammalian brain. *Proc. Natl. Acad. Sci. U S A.* 1996; 93: 14895-900.

El Maarouf A, Petridis AK, Rutishauser U. Use of polysialic acid in repair of the central nervous system. *Proc. Natl. Acad. Sci. USA* 2006; 103: 16989-94.

Fujimoto I, Bruses JL, Rutishauser U. 2001. Regulation of cell adhesion by polysi- alic acid. Effects on cadherin, immuno- globulin cell adhesion molecule, and integrin function and independence from neural cell adhesion molecule binding or signaling activity. *J. Biol. Chem.* 276: 31745-31751.

Glüer S, Schelp C, von Schweinitz D, Gerardy-Schahn R. Polysialylated neural cell adhesion molecule in childhood rhabdomyosarcoma. *Pediatr. Res.* 1998; 43:145-7.

Hu H, Tomasiewicz H, Magnuson T, Rutishauser U. The role of polysialic acid in migration of olfactory bulb interneuron precursors in the subventricular zone. *Neuron* 1996; 16: 735-43.

Hoffman S, Sorkin BC, White PC, Brackenbury R, Mailhammer R, Rutishauser U, Cunningham BA, Edelman GM. Chemical characterization of a neural cell adhesion molecule purified from embryonic brain membranes. *J. Biol. Chem.* 1982; 257: 7720-29.

Miyahara R, Tanaka F, Nakagawa T, Matsuoka K, Isii K, Wada H. Expression of neural cell adhesion molecules (polysialylated form of neural cell adhesion molecule and L1-cell adhesion molecule) on resected small cell lung cancer specimens: in relation to proliferation state. *J. Surg. Oncol.* 2001; 77:49-54.

Ono K, Tomasiewicz H, Magnuson T, Rutishauser U. N-CAM mutation inhibits tangential neuronal migration and is phenocopied by enzymatic removal of polysialic acid. *Neuron* 1994; 13:595-609.

Johnson CP, Fujimoto I, Rutishauser U, Leckband DE. Direct evidence that neural cell adhesion molecule (NCAM) polysialylation increases intermembrane repulsion and abrogates adhesion. *J. Biol. Chem.* 2005; 280:137-45.

Petridis AK, Wedderkopp H, Hugo HH, Maximilian Mehdorn H. Polysialic acid overexpression in malignant astrocytomas. *Acta Neurochir.* (Wien) 2009; 151:601-3.

Petridis AK, El-Maarouf A, Rutishauser U. Polysialic acid regulates cell contact-dependent neuronal differentiation of progenitor cells from the subventricular zone. *Dev. Dyn.* 2004; 230:675-84.

Seidenfaden R, Krauter A, Schertzinger F et al. Polysialic acid directs tumor cell growth by controlling heterophilic neural cell adhesion molecule interactions. *Mol. Cell Biol.* 2003; 23:5908-18.

Suzuki M, Suzuki M, Nakayama J, Suzuki A, Angata K, Chen S, Sakai K, Hagihara K, Yamaguchi Y, Fukuda M. Polysialic acid facilitates tumor invasion by glioma cells. *Glycobiology*. 2005; 15:887-94.

In: Recent Advances in Adhesions Research   ISBN: 978-1-62417-447-6
Editors: A. McFarland and M. Akins   © 2013 Nova Science Publishers, Inc.

Chapter 6

IMPLICATION OF POLYSIALIC ACID OVEREXPRESSION ON TUMORIGENESIS OF NEUROECTODERMAL AND OTHER TUMORS: IMPAIRMENT OF CELL ADHESION

Athanasios K. Petridis[*]
Wedau Kliniken, Duisburg, Germany
University Hospital Schleswig-Holstein, Kiel, Germany

ABSTRACT

Polysialic Acid is a carbohydrate, which binds to the neural cell adhesion molecule NCAM, and contains a high amount of water. It is known that polysialic acid attenuates cell-cell interactions and inhibits differentiation as well as enhances cell migration. Both features are characteristics of highly malignant cancer cells. It has been shown that in a number of highly malignant tumors like glioblastomas, rhabdomyosarcomas, neuroblastomas, and small cell lung cancer, polysialic acid is over-expressed on the surface of these tumor cells. In the present review the possible benefit of polysialic acid overexpression for the tumor cells is discussed, as well as diagnostic and therapeutic strategies towards polysialic acid.

[*] Corresponding author. Neurosurgical Department, Wedau Kliniken Duisburg, Zu den Rehwiesen 9-11, 47055 Duisburg, Germany. E-mail: opticdisc@aol.com.

Keywords: Polysialic acid, neuroectodermal tumors, CSF

INTRODUCTION

Polysialic Acid (PSA) is a carbohydrate, which is largely hydrated and enhances cell migration of neural progenitor cells from the subventricular zone to the olfactory bulb [1-6]. On the other hand, it is known that PSA acts as a negative regulator of cell-cell interactions and prevents progenitor cells in the central nervous system (CNS) to differentiate prematurely [7-9]. When progenitor cells reach their destiny, PSA is downregulated, migration stops and differentiation into olfactory bulb neurons begins [8].

Additionally to the physiological expression of PSA it could be shown that PSA is also overexpressed in a number of neuroectodermal tumors and some other carcinomas which are highly malignant, highly invasive and metastatic. The role of PSA expression in these malignant tumors and a preview of a therapeutic potential through PSA cleavage is discussed in the present article.

MATERIAL AND METHODS

Pubmed search was conducted for polysialic acid and tumors and polysialic acid and cancer. The search gave 158 hits. The review is based on the literature search as well as the observations made in the authors publications, which are cited in the present work.

DISCUSSION

Polysialic Acid Overexpression in Tumor Cells

It does not surprise that PSA is overexpressed in a number of malignant cells since it helps to keep cells away from the "cellular social network". In other words it is acting as a factor of antisocialising cancer cells and makes them act as" anarchistic cells" in the cellular community of the organism. Neuroblastoma cells, as well as glioblastoma cells among others overexpress PSA [7,9,10,11].

PSA overexpression in neuroblastoma cells showed a positive correlation with metastasis [12]. In pituitary tumors the expression of PSA correlated with an extrasellar invasion of the tumors [13, 14].

PSA positive non small cell lung cancer cells correlate with a significant worse prognosis [15].

The re-expression of PSA in Wilm´s tumor had lead to considering PSA as an oncodevelopmental antigen [16]. As expected it has been postulated that PSA weakens NCAM –NCAM cell adhesion and increases cancer cell detachment, therefore inducing metastasis. The body immune response can also become negatively modulated by PSA overexpression since it can mask and hide tumor-specific antigens [17]. Tumor cells can use the expression of PSA to escape the immune-system. In pancreatic tumor cells a positive correlation of PSA over-expression and tumor cell proliferation could be shown and neural invasion of pancreatic tumor cells (correlating with the worse prognosis) was associated with PSA overexpression on these tumor cells [18].

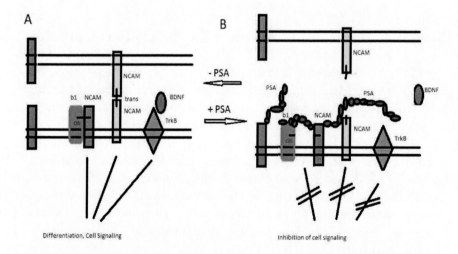

Figure 1. A.Without PSA cells are able to interact through trans-signaling. Cooperation between molecules on the membrane of the same cell is possible and physiologic signaling cascades can be initiated. Neurotrophic factors activate their specific receptors like BDNF and its TrkB receptor. B. When PSA is expressed trans- and cis – interactions are inhibited. Neurotrophic receptors can blocked and cells lose almost every contact to their environment. Cleavage of PSA with endo N could re-establish the interactions of cells and lead the cells to physiological signaling cascades.

Polysialic Acid Detection Could be Used As a Prognostic Marker

As already mentioned, overexpression of PSA is a negative prognostic factor in cancer. Highly invasive tumors over-express PSA. PSA-NCAM enzyme-linked-immunosorbent assay (ELISA) for detection of PSA in the cerebrospinal fluid (CSF), showed that PSA was a reliable marker to predict a more aggressive, metastatic and invasive medulloblastoma. PSA in the CSF could be detected in refractory cases even when CSF-cytology and imaging failed [19]. In another study serum levels of PSA-NCAM detected by immunoluminescence showed a significant (6-fold) increase of PSA-NCAM in children with advanced stage of neuroblastoma [20]. In the mentioned studies it is showed that PSA-detection is an excellent marker for the identification of aggressive tumors in the serum and the CSF. Immunohistochemically PSA can easily be detected by different antibodies and identify a very aggressive tumor like highly invasive neuroectodermal tumors, medullary thyroid tumors, rhabdomyosarcomas just to mention some [21-23].

Molecular Mechanisms Involving PSA-NCAM Overexpression

Pax3 is a transcription factor that is in involved in Oncogenesis. It has been showed that transfection with Pax3 into a human medulloblastoma cell line increases NCAM polysialylation [24]. Gain of function mutations in Pax3 caused cancer in human cell lines and a chimeric transcription factor PAX3-FKHR, produced by a chromosomal translocation in cancer could regulate an overexpression of PSA-NCAM [25]. Another study showed that beta1-integrin as well as NCAM are associated with neurite outgrowth and differentiation of neuroblastoma cells. NCAM and beta1-integrin interact on the cell surface and the PSA overexpression on NCAM inhibits the interaction of both molecules rendering both molecules inactive and blocking differentiation of neuroblastoma cells [26].

This finding is in so far important because it shows that PSA is not only inhibiting cell-cell interaction but also interactions between molecules on the membrane of the same cell. Trans- and cis- interactions can be inhibited, which can lead to a complete deregulation of cellular signaling pathways. On the other hand neurotrophic factors like Brain Derived Neurotrophic Factor (BDNF) are not able to activate their receptors through the masking of such receptors through PSA [27, 28]. PSA seems to block in general a huge amount of cell interactions with the environment.

Therapeutic Approach through PSA-Cleavage

Endoneuraminidase N (endo N) is a PSA specific cleavage enzyme with no proven adverse effects. The treatment of PSA-expressing neuroblastoma cells with endo N showed the initiation of differentiation of the neuroblastoma cells and the inhibition of their migratory potential [8, 9].

Intrathecal application of endo N removed PSA from subventricular zone progenitors showing that the intrathecal application of endo N could reach a possible target into the CNS [8].

Unfortunatelly the application of endo N into the blood seems to be inefficient for removal of PSA in tumor cells since endo N is immediately inactivated by the blood (own observations).

REFERENCES

Ono K, Tomasiewicz H, Magnuson T, Rutishauser U (1994). NCAM mutation inhibits tangential neuronal migartion and is phenocopied by enzymatic removal of polysialic acid. *Neuron* 13: 595-609.

Doetsch F and Alvarez-Buylla A (1996). Network of tangential pathways for neuronal migration in adult mammalian brain. *Proc Natl Acad Sci* USA 93: 14895-14900.

Hu H, Tomasiewicz H, Magnuson T, Rutishauser U (1996). *The role of polysialic acid in migration of olfactory bulb interneuron precursors in the subventricular zone.*

Tomasiewicz H, Ono K, Yee D, Thompson C, Goridis C, Rutishauser U, Magnuson T (1993). Genetic deletion of a neural cell adhesion molecule variant (NCAM-180) produces distinct defects in the central nervous system. *Neuron* 11: 1163-1174.

Cremer H, Lange R, Christoph A, Plomann M, Vopper G, Roes J, Brown R, Baldwin S, Kraemer P, Scheff S (1994). Inactivation of the NCAM gene in mice results in size reduction of the olfactory bulb and deficits in spatial learning. *Nature* 367: 455-459.

Chazal G, Durbec P, Jankowski A, Rougon G, Cremer H (2000). Consequences of neural cell adhesion molecule deficiency on cell migration in the rostral migratory stream of the mouse. *J Neurosci* 20: 1446-1457.

Rutishauser U (1998). Polysialic acid at the cell surface: biophysics in service of cell interactions and tissue plasticity. *J. Cell Biochem* 70: 304-312.

Petridis AK, El Maarouf A, Rutishauser U (2004). Polysialic acid regulates cell contact-dependent neuronal differentiation of progenitor cells from the subventricular zone. *Develop Dyn* 230: 675-684.

Seidenfaden R, Krauter A, Schertzinger F, Gerardy-Schahn R, Hildebrandt H (2003). Polysialic acid directs tumor cell growth by controlling heterophilic neural cell adhesion molecule interactions. *Mol Cell Biol* 23: 5908-5918.

Suzuki M, Suzuki M, Nakayama J, Suzuki A, Angata K, Chen S, Sakai K, Hagihara K, Yamaguchi Y, Fukuda M (2005). Polysialic acid facilitates tumor invasion by glioma cells. *Glycobiology* 15: 887-894.

Petridis AK, Wedderkopp H, Hugo HH, Mehdorn HM (2009). Polysialic acid overexpression in malignant astrocytomas. *Acta Neurochir* 151: 601-604.

Valentiner U, Mühlenhoff M, Lehmann U, Hildebrandt H, Schumacher U (2011). Expression oft he neural cell adhesion molecule and polysialic acid in human neuroblastoma cell lines. *Int J Oncol* 39: 417-424.

Trouillas J, Daniel L, Guigard M-P, Tong S, Gouvernet J, Jouanneau E, Jan M, Perrin G, Fischer G, Tabarin A, Rougon G, Figarella-Branger D (2003). Polysialylated neural cell adhesion molecules expressed in human pituitary tumors and related to extrasellar invasion. *J Neurosurg* 98: 1084-1093.

Wierinckx A, Auger C, Devauchelle P, Reynaud A, Chevallier P, Jan M, Perrin G, Fevre-Montange M, Rey C, Figarella-Branger D, Raverot G, Belin M-F, Lachuer J, Trouillas J (2007). A diagnostic marker set for invasion, proliferation, and aggressiveness of prolactin pituitary tumors. *Endocrine-related Cancer* 14: 887-900.

Tanaka F, Otake Y, Nakagawa T, Kawano Y, Miyahara R, Li M, Yanagihara K, Inui K, Oyanagi H, Yamada T, Nakayama J, Fujimoto I, Ikenaka K, Wada H (2001). Prognostic significance of polysialic acid expression in resected non-small cell lung cancer. *Cancer Research 61:* 1666-1670.

Roth J, Zuber C, Wagner P, Taatjes DJ, Weisgerber C, Heitz PU, Goridis C, Bitter-Suermann D (1988). Presence of long chain form of polysialic acid oft he neural adhesion molecule in Wilm's tumor. *Am J Pathol* 133: 227-239.

Bitter-Suermann (1993). Influence of bacterlial polysialic capsules on host defence: masquerade and mimicry, in : J. Roth, U. Rutishauser, F. Troy II (eds.). *Polysialic acid: From microbes to man,* Birkhauser, Basel: 11.

Kameda K, Shimada H, Ishikawa T, Takimoto A, Momiyama N, Hasegawa S, Misuta K, Nakano A, Nagashima Y, Ichikawa Y (1999). Expression of highly polysialylatde neural cell adhesion molecule in pancreatic cancer neural invasive lesion. *Cancer Letter* 137: 201-207.

Dubois C, Figarella-Branger D, Rougon G, Rampini C (1998).Polysialylated NCAM in CSF, a marker for invasive medulloblastoma. *C R Seanes Soc Biol Fil* 192: 289-296. French.

Glüer S, Schelp C, Madry N, von Schweinitz D, Eckhardt M, Gerardy-Schahn R (1998). Serum polysialylated neural cell adhesion molecule in childhood neuroblastoma. *British J of Cancer* 78: 106-110.

Komminoth P, Roth J, Saremaslani P, Matias_Guiu X, Wolfe HJ, Heitz PU. (1994). Polysialic acid of the neural cell adhesion molecule in the human thyroid: a marker for medullary thyroid carcinoma and primary C-cell hyperplasia. An immunohistochemical study on 79 thyroid lesions. *Am J Surg Pathol* 18: 399-411.

Glüer S, Schelp C, von Schweinitz D, Gerardy-Schahn R (1998). Polysialylated neural cell adhesion molecule in childhood rhabdomyosarcoma. *Pediatr Res* 43: 145-147.

Glüer S, Schelp C, Gerardy-Schahn R, von Schweinitz D (1998). Polysialylated neural cell adhesion molecule as a marker for differential diagnosis in pediatric tumors. *J Pediatr Surg* 33: 1516-1520.

Mayanil CSK, George D, Mania-Farnell B, Bremer CL, McLone D, Bremer EG (2000). Overexpression of murine Pax3 increases NCAM polysialylation in a human medulloblastoma cell line. *J Biol Chem* 275: 23259-23266.

Ginsberg JP, Davis RJ, Bennicelli JL, Nauta LE, Barr FG (1998). Up-regulation of MET but not neural cell adhesion molecule expression by the PAX3-FKHR fusion protein in alveolar rhabdomyosarcoma. *Cancer Res* 58: 3542-3546.

Petridis AK, Nikolopoulos SN, El-Maarouf A (2011). Physical and functional cooperation of neural cell adhesion molecule and beta1-integrin in neurite outgrowth induction. *J Clin Neurosci* 18: 1109-1113.

Petridis AK, El-Maarouf A (2011). Brain-derived neurotrophic factor levels influence the balance of migration and differentiation of subventricular zone cells, but not guidance to the olfactory bulb. *J Clin Neurosci.* 18: 265-270.

Muller D, Djebbara-Hannas Z, Jourdain P, Vutskits L, Durbec P, Rougon G, Kiss JZ (2000). Brain-derived neurotrophic factor restores long-term potentiation in polysialic acid-neural cell adhesion molecule-deficient hippocampus. *Proc Natl Acad Sci* USA 97: 4315-4320.

In: Recent Advances in Adhesions Research   ISBN: 978-1-62417-447-6
Editors: A. McFarland and M. Akins   © 2013 Nova Science Publishers, Inc.

Chapter 7

EFFECTS OF ANTI-CELL ADHESION MOLECULES TO PREVENT HEART TRANSPLANT REJECTION

Jun-ichi Suzuki[1], Masahito Ogawa[1], Yasunobu Hirata[1], Ryozo Nagai[2] and Mitsuaki Isobe[3]*

Departments of [1]Advanced Clinical Science and Therapeutics,
[2]Cardiovascular Medicine, University of Tokyo, Japan
[3]Department of Cardiovascular Medicine,
Tokyo Medical and Dental University, Japan

ABSTRACT

Although 100,000 cardiac transplants have been performed, rejection is still a serious problem. Several adhesion molecules play a critical role in the progression of rejection. Recent investigations have proved some promising methodologies targeting cell adhesion molecules for preventing or treating inflammatory diseases. Although neutralizing antibodies are known to be an effective treatment in cardiovascular diseases, their effect on cardiac transplantation is to be elucidated. In this

* Correspondence to: Jun-ichi Suzuki, Department of Advanced Clinical Science and Therapeutics, Graduate School of Medicine, University of Tokyo, 7-3-1 Hongo, Bunkyo, Tokyo 113-8655, Japan; phone 81-3-5800-9116, fax 81-3-5800-9182, e-mail junichisuzuki-circ@umin.ac.jp.

review article, we described some promising methodologies that use blocking cell adhesion molecules to prevent cardiac rejection.

Keywords: heart transplant; chronic rejection; vasculopathy; inflammation; antibody; immunoglobulin

1. INTRODUCTION

Cardiac transplantation is a common surgical procedure; almost 100,000 heart transplantations have been performed worldwide [1]. However, coronary allograft vasculopathy (CAV), which is a phenomenon of chronic rejection, is still a serious problem [2]. Because CAV involves the entire allograft arteries, conservative treatments, such as angioplasty or bypass grafting, are not practical. Therefore, CAV is the biggest problem against the prognosis in the heart transplant recipients [3]. Several adhesion molecules promote rejection; CAV is characterized by intimal thickening comprised of proliferative smooth muscle cells (SMCs) and extracellular matrix (ECM). In early stages, there is a subendothelial accumulation of mononuclear cell infiltration associated with markers of endothelial cell (EC) activation. Because endothelial or perivascular cellular immune injury induce persistent allograft vascular damage, inflammatory cells and activated ECs secrete adhesion molecule to recruit and activate SMCs [4]. This review article describes the possibilities the anti-adhesion molecules to prevent CAV.

2. ANTI-ICAM-1 AND LFA-1

We found that anti-intercellular adhesion molecule-1 (ICAM-1) and anti-lymphocyte function-associated antigen-1 (LFA-1) antibodies (Abs) induce immunologic tolerance in murine heart transplantation [5]. To clarify the mechanism of tolerance induction by an ICAM-1 and LFA-1 blockade, we characterized the cytokine profiles. Production and transcription of Th2 cytokines were enhanced in the mice treated with the mAbs, whereas Th1 cytokines were suppressed. Of note, exogenous IL-2 administration prevented the induction of tolerance to cardiac allografts [6]. Mixed lymphocyte reaction showed that splenocytes from allograft recipients treated with the mAbs showed normal allogeneic response [7]. However, the effect of mAb blockade on CAV had yet to be elucidated at that time. To evaluate the effects of anti-

ICAM-1 plus anti-LFA-1 mAbs in preventing CAV, we treated C3H/He mice that received BALB/c mice hearts with anti-ICAM-1 plus anti-LFA-1 mAbs for the first 5 days after transplantation. For control studies, FK506 was administered daily to other allograft recipients. We revealed that the allografts from mice that received FK506 treatment showed heavy neointimal thickening with increased expression of ICAM-1 and vascular cell adhesion molecule (VCAM)-1. Conversely, anti-ICAM-1 plus anti-LFA-1 mAbs showed almost no CAV development [8]. Thus, we clarified that a short-term blockade of ICAM-1 and LFA-1 adhesion not only induced immunologic tolerance to cardiac allografts but also prevented CAV through altered expression of cytokines.

3. ANTI-VCAM-1 AND VLA-4

Other cell adhesion molecules, VCAM-1 and very late antigen (VLA)-4, play a critical role in cellular immunologic activation. It was reported that anti-VCAM-1 mAb plus anti-VLA-4 mAb administration prolonged graft survival, however, the blockade leads to tolerance only in some cases. To reveal the different immunological mechanism, we transplanted BALB/c mice hearts into C3H recipients. Anti-VCAM-1 plus anti-VLA-4 mAbs or anti-ICAM-1 plus anti-LFA-1 mAbs was administered for 5 days. For control study, a third group of mice received daily administration of FK506. The cardiac allografts and recipient spleens were harvested on day 7; the expression of cytokines were detected. We revealed that Th2 cytokines (IL-4 and IL-l0) were markedly enhanced and Th1 cytokines (IFN-gamma and IL-2) were suppressed in recipients treated with anti-ICAM-1 mAb plus anti-LFA-1 mAb. However, poor Th2 cytokine expression allowed persistent Th1 cytokine expression in recipient mice with anti-VCAM-1 mAb plus anti-VLA-4 mAb treatment. Both Th1 and Th2 cytokine expression was suppressed in FK506-treated mice. We concluded that immunological tolerance and prolonged graft survival induced by blocking cell adhesion is regulated by different cytokine expression [9].

4. ANTI-SELECTINS

Selectins play an important role in the inflammatory response by eliciting leukocyte rolling. The roles of E- and P-selectins in the acute rejection of cardiac allografts remain unclear. Thus, to evaluate whether E- and P-selectins participate in the pathophysiology of heart rejection, heterotopic heart transplantation was performed in both mice and rats. Immunohistochemistry, flow-cytometry, and RT-PCR were performed to evaluate E-, P-selectin and sialyl Lewis X (SLeX) expression in rejected cardiac allografts. The effects of short-term administration of mAbs to E- and P-selectins on cardiac allograft survival were also evaluated. We demonstrated that significant prolongation of graft survival was observed in mice treated with either anti-E- or P-selectin mAbs, or both. The enhanced endothelial and mRNA expression of E- and P-selectins was observed in the rejected cardiac allografts. Some graft infiltrating mononuclear cells were double-stained with both anti-SLeX and anti-alphabetaT cell receptor mAbs. Flow-cytometric analysis of graft-infiltrating cells also showed enhanced SLeX expression. We concluded that both P- and E-selectins are critically involved in the early development of acute heart rejection [10].

5. INHIBITION OF ICOS

A costimulatory molecule, inducible co-stimulator (ICOS), was identified as the third member of the CD28 family [11]. ICOS is expressed on T cell surfaces after activation, and it causes T cell proliferation [12]. A role for ICOS in cardiac allograft rejection has also been reported [13]; blockade of the ICOS pathway prolonged cardiac allograft survival in a murine heart transplant model. Cyclosporine A in conjunction with anti-ICOS therapy induced permanent allograft survival; however, immunologic tolerance was not confirmed in the model. Recently, we demonstrated the effect of blockade of the ICOS and costimulatory pathways in murine cardiac transplantation. ICOS was strongly expressed in association with cardiac allograft rejection. The combined treatment with ICOSIg plus cytotoxic T-lymphocyte antigen 4 (CTLA4) Ig prolonged allograft survival, leading to donor-specific tolerance. In this model, CAV was significantly reduced after treatment with ICOSIg plus CTLA4Ig compared to treatment with tacrolimus. In vitro study showed that CTLA4Ig suppressed T cell proliferation in a dose-dependent manner. Although modest reduction in proliferation was observed with the single treatment, the combined therapy with ICOSIg plus CTLA4Ig suppressed T cell proliferation. Thus, we concluded that ICOS could be another regulator in T cell activation that leads to acute and chronic cardiac allograft rejection.

Blockade of the ICOS pathway with anti-ICOS antibody or ICOSIg may have therapeutic potential on CAV [14].

CONCLUSION

Although improved immunosuppressants have resulted in reduced acute rejection rates, CAV is a problem yet to be resolved [2]. Because the number of heart transplants has decreased [1], preventing CAV is critical for long-term prognosis of heart transplant recipients. Further studies are needed to clarify the clinical usefulness of blocking adhesion molecules for the prevention of CAV.

REFERENCES

[1]   Stehlik J, Edwards LB, Kucheryavaya AY, et al. The Registry of the International Society for Heart and Lung Transplantation: Twenty-eighth Adult Heart Transplant Report--2011. *J. Heart Lung Transplant.* 2011; 30: 1078-94.

[2]   Suzuki J, Isobe M, Morishita R, et al. Characteristics of chronic rejection in heart transplantation –Important elements of pathogenesis and future treatments-. *Circ. J.* 2010; 74: 233-9.

[3]   Mitchell RN. Graft vascular disease: immune response meets the vessel wall. *Annu. Rev. Pathol.* 2009; 4: 19-47.

[4]   Mitchell RN, Libby P. Vascular remodeling in transplant vasculopathy. *Circ. Res.* 2007; 100: 967–78.

[5]   Isobe M, Yagita H, Okumura K, et al. Specific acceptance of cardiac allograft after treatment with antibodies to ICAM-1 and LFA-1. *Science* 1992; 255: 1125-7.

[6]   Isobe M, Suzuki J, Yamazaki S, et al. Regulation by differential development of Th1 and Th2 cells in peripheral tolerance to cardiac allograft induced by blocking ICAM-1/LFA-1 adhesion. *Circulation* 1997; 96: 2247-53.

[7]   Isobe M, Suzuki J, Yamazaki S, et al. Assessment of tolerance induction to cardiac allograft by anti-ICAM-1 and anti-LFA-1 monoclonal antibodies. *J. Heart Lung Transplant.* 1997; 16: 1149-56.

[8]   Suzuki J, Isobe M, Yamazaki S, et al. Inhibition of accelerated coronary atherosclerosis with short-term blockade of intercellular adhesion molecule-1 and lymphocyte function-associated antigen-1 in a heterotopic murine model of heart transplantation. *J. Heart Lung Transplant.* 1997; 16: 1141-48.

[9]   Suzuki J, Isobe M, Izawa A, et al. Differential Th1 and Th2 cell regulation of murine cardiac allograft acceptance by blocking cell adhesion of ICAM-1/LFA-1 and VCAM-1/VLA-4. *Transplant. Immunol.* 1999; 7: 65-72.

[10] Yamazaki S, Isobe M, Suzuki J, et al. Role of selectin-dependent adhesion in cardiac allograft rejection. *J. Heart and Lung Transplant.* 1998; 17: 1007-16.

[11] Hutloff A, Dittrich AM, Beier KC, et al. ICOS is an inducible T-cell co-stimulator structurally and functionally related to CD28. *Nature* 1999; 397: 263-6.

[12] Yoshinaga SK, Whoriskey JS, Khare SD, et al. T-cell co-stimulation through B7RP-1 and ICOS. *Nature* 1999; 402: 827-32.

[13] Ozkaynak E, Gao W, Shemmeri N, et al. Importance of ICOS-B7RP-1 costimulation in acute and chronic allograft rejection. *Nat. Immunol.* 2001; 2: 591–6.

[14] Kosuge H, Suzuki J, Haraguchi G, et al. Critical role of inducible costimulator signaling in the development of arteriosclerosis. *Arterioscler. Thromb. Vasc. Biol.* 2006; 26: 2660-5.

INDEX

D

E

F

O

P

Q

R